MUSIC
IN GERIATRIC CARE

Ruth Bright

Music Therapist, New South Wales Department of Health

MAGNAMUSIC-BATON, INC.
10370 PAGE INDUSTRIAL BLVD.
ST. LOUIS, MO. 63132

First published in 1972 by

ANGUS AND ROBERTSON (PUBLISHERS) PTY LTD

National Library of Australia card number and ISBN hard bound edition 0 207 12416 7

This paperback edition issued in 1980 by Musicgraphics for the world.

MUSIC
IN GERIATRIC CARE

The use of music in geriatric care is less well established than in the field of psychiatry — this book describes Ruth Bright's success as a working music therapist in the use of music in the care and rehabilitation of the aged. She sees music as providing an emotive quality often lacking in medical treatment, whether physical or psychological, which gives each individual a chance to express himself as a person, not simply a patient.

By providing the opportunity for shared interest and activity, music can assist in the socialization of the elderly within social clubs and hospitals. The associative powers of music can build a happy atmosphere in group work and help to overcome the feelings of confusion, loss and inadequacy so unfortunately common among the elderly. Musical activity is useful in improving motivation and reinforcing the learning of exercises in physical therapy involving the re-learning of motor skills or the learning of new skills to compensate for loss or impairment.

This book is more than a theoretical treatise: it gives practical suggestions for planning musical programs, as an adjunct to social work and to medical and paramedical disciplines, and as a therapeutic activity in its own right. It will be of the greatest use in all the helping professions.

Because music can enter so many aspects of treatment, the author emphasizes its importance as a cohesive factor, assisting in the total medical and paramedical treatment of a patient who is subject to the attention of many different specialists.

Foreword

At first sight the title may seem to be rather a restricting one and the field limited. However, Mrs Ruth Bright has demonstrated in this important book that music in the care of geriatric patients is an essential part of the total therapeutic approach. In modern times, with the advent of specialisation, the individual tends to be forgotten and his illness becomes the important factor. It is thus all too easy to be fascinated by curing of the patient's physical complaint while ignoring his mental health. No one reading this book can fail to be impressed by the usefulness of music in a general cohesive way and also in the special application of music, as for instance in the treatment of aphasia. This little volume contains much more however than the bare outline of the use of music in the care of elderly ill people. The whole concept of music in therapy and much interesting information on the mental health of the elderly and the ultimate aim of treatment, are among the topics clearly described.

The facts put forward leave the reader in no doubt that music therapy must be taken seriously and that it has an important part to play, in combination with psychotherapy, with physiotherapy and with speech therapy, in the ultimate cure of many older people. In the section on practical considerations, much thought has been given to the application of the theoretical discussions put forward in the previous section. Practical and worthwhile advice is given on equipment and staffing problems and the book is well illustrated to show what can be done, in individual cases, and in group therapy, to improve the care of patients.

There is no doubt that the points and issues discussed in the pages to follow will be of immense value to all those interested in the elderly. They will give the doctor much information on the practical procedures which can help the morale and mental health of his older patients. The physiotherapist, speech therapist, occupational therapist, social worker and chiropodist, will all benefit from the advice and thoughts contained herein. Older people themselves will be encouraged and stimulated by the amount of careful consideration that has gone into the factors concerned with their health and with keeping them fit.

In order to complete this study, there is one most important chapter on contraindications to music therapy and these are clearly put forward—examples includes musicogenic epilepsy and boredom or dislike of music, while the problem of emotional disturbance is also noted and over-sensitivity to noise is also rightly mentioned as a contraindication.

It has always been my belief that we are only at the beginning of our understanding of how to treat the elderly sick and this important and valuable book does add one more step to our knowledge of the handling of those who are ill and old.

I am very proud indeed to have been asked to write this foreword and I am certain that the condition of many many older people will be improved as a result of the methods here recorded.

L. Ferguson Anderson, O.B.E., C.ST.J., M.D., F.R.C.P.
David Cargill Professor of Geriatric Medicine,
The University, Glasgow.
May 1972.

Contents

Introduction

Geriatrics and its partner gerontology constitute a fast developing area of endeavour, but so far music in the geriatric care of patients is less well established than in the psychiatric field—although some of the practical social uses of music have been recognized for many years, and work with psychogeriatric patients has been described.

Today the trend in medical care is towards the total care approach. However, because of the specialization of different aspects of treatment—specialist services (such as orthopaedics, neurology, pathology), physiotherapy, speech therapy, occupational therapy and social work—it is sometimes difficult to achieve such a unified approach, and patients are treated in 'bits and pieces' instead of as whole persons. There is too little in common between the different aspects of treatment for there to be any feeling of unity to the patient. Furthermore, it is all too easy for the therapist to lose sight of the patient as a person, forgetting the emotional turmoil into which he has been thrown by the illness itself, or—in having to learn old skills in a new way—by the processes of rehabilitation.

In these problems, music can help. Because it can enter into so many aspects of treatment, music can act as a cohesive force, binding together the diversity of medical and paramedical treatment.

In most musical activities, the patient has some degree of choice in what is done—the songs which are sung, the music to be discussed. For many ageing people, such opportunities for choice are narrowly confined. The work done in physiotherapy, although undeniably for the patient's good, is often difficult and even painful, but it must be done. The same may be true of other aspects of treatment—e.g. diet is often restricted, and even when the reasons for the restrictions are explained, this does not make the food any more enjoyable. For patients in a nursing home, even a good one, the routine of life is necessarily fairly rigid, even to the time of waking and sleeping, the time television is turned on and the programs which are shown.

These factors, added to those imposed by advancing age and by disability, may add up to an unbearable sense of restraint and frustration, and the patient is left wondering what he can decide for himself. The social worker, of course, takes cognizance of such problems, but few nursing homes or geriatric units have a full-time worker, and many are not able to have even part-time assistance in this regard. Nevertheless, there is usually someone who can arrange a 'skeleton' program of musical activities.

This is essential, because music gives to our work, whether in physical or psychological medicine, the emotive quality which is so often lacking, providing each individual with the chance to express himself as a *person* and not just as 'the patient'.

It seems relevant to state here the author's personal creed of geriatrics, the point of view which colours all the discussion of the many topics which make up this book. Each of us presumably has a slightly different outlook, determined by our own disciplines. Through the eyes of a musician, who also has general interests in the problems of humanity, geriatrics is seen as concerning:

The body, in

1. maintaining and improving existing levels of physical fitness,
2. minimizing effects of existing illness,
3. preventing development of further disability.

The mind and the spirit, in

1. maintaining the patient's status as an individual,
2. minimizing the adverse effects of age and disability by helping patients with the emotional and intellectual difficulties of disability and their changing status in the community, and thus
3. preventing mental and emotional disability.

The community, in

1. greater orientation towards age and maturity and away from excessive orientation towards youth,

2. greater understanding of problems of ageing and disability, eliminating both rejection and over-protection,

3. educating people to make use of existing services, and—like Oliver Twist—to ask for more and better services.

This philosophy has greatly influenced the writing of this book. It will be noticed that many of the subjects contained herein are not strictly confined to music as such, but enter briefly into such matters as group psychology, learning and motivation, and the physical treatment of certain conditions. The intention is not thereby to offer an authoritative volume in geriatric rehabilitation, but to substantiate the author's beliefs that one works more intelligently and more productively when one understands something of the physiological mechanisms underlying health and disease, and of the psychological, physical and emotional problems of each patient.

The various topics have been arranged as systematically as possible, and, where there is unavoidable overlapping, references will be found so that—with the index for additional guidance—there should be little difficulty in finding details required.

Grateful acknowledgment is given for the help of many geriatricians and other specialists who have allowed me to visit their departments, and who have given generously their time in guiding my work in hospitals as well as in the writing of this book. Mention must be made of the invaluable help given by librarians of the Health Department of New South Wales in finding the many books and references needed.

Thanks are also due to the many physiotherapists from several rehabilitation units who devised and supervised the various programs of group work which are described, some of which are illustrated herein; to the hospital authorities and patients who gave permission for the photographs to be taken; and to Dawn Wood for her help with the illustrations.

I especially wish to thank Dr Richard B. Geeves, M.B., B.S., F.R.A.C.G.P., who has given so much help in my studies of geriatric rehabilitation.

R.B.

March 1972

THEORETICAL
CONSIDERATIONS

1. *History*

As has been described elsewhere,[1] the concept of music-in-therapy
dates back to the eighteenth century, with occasional writings
(on both the physical and psychological effects of music) since
then. But it was not until after the 1914-1918 war, when the
occurrence of great numbers of cases of 'shell-shock' made new
approaches to psychiatric medicine necessary, that music therapy
received any great emphasis. Today, professional training is available in the United Kingdom, Germany and the United States.
Music therapists are employed in hundreds of hospitals and there
is continual publication of results of research and clinical experience in the professional journals[2] devoted to music therapy. The
subjects dealt with cover a diverse range of work with music—
in social work, cerebral palsy, for children with multiple handicaps, for autistic children, behaviour modification by behaviourist
techniques employing music for reinforcement, for 'thalidomide
children' and for slow learners, as well as the more obvious applications in psychiatric hospitals.

The training available in the U.K. is not identical with that in
either Germany or the U.S.A. (where music therapy is available
as a bachelor's degree, a master's degree, and at doctorate level at
many universities), but yet there is unity in outlook of the training schemes in that they are concerned with the 'whole man', and,
by using different musically oriented techniques, set out to help
patients to a happier and healthier way of life.

There are still people who see music as an entertainment, having therapeutic value only in a recreational sense, but such views
are declining and it is clear that the time is not far distant when
music therapy will be as generally accepted as a form of treatment
as are occupational, speech and physical therapy.

How soon training will be available in all major centres is not
known, but even when courses are established everywhere, there

will still be small hospitals, nursing homes and other organizations where it will not be possible to employ a music therapist. Thus, for some time to come, there will be a place for the amateur, or the musically-minded from other disciplines, to organize musical activities which have a therapeutic aim.

The study of ageing is now receiving considerable emphasis throughout the world, and conferences are held regularly in many different centres. At these, there is discussion not only of the physiological aspects of ageing and its day-to-day manifestations, but also of loneliness, motivation, socializing influences, the care of those for whom rehabilitation proves impossible, and the other problems which concern us. For a significant proportion of these, music has an answer.

It is hoped that this book will provide guidelines and ideas for the establishment of a program of musical activities, not making hard and fast rules but offering suggestions which can then be developed according to the circumstances—the type of patients, the musical resources of the staff, and the amount of time available. The history of music therapy has just begun, and each of us has the opportunity of adding another page or another chapter.

REFERENCES
1. Bright, R. *Music and Mental Health: An Introduction to Music Therapy in Australia*, N.S.W. Dept. of Health, Sydney, 1967. (Chapter 1).
2. *British Journal of Music Therapy*, pub. quarterly by the British Society for Music Therapy, London. *Journal of Music Therapy*, pub. quarterly by the National Association for Music Therapy Inc. Kansas, U.S.A.

2. *Music as a socialising and preventive measure*

Isolation is a common phenomenon among the ageing population, and for many it is the cause of grave loneliness and depression. For some, severe guilt feelings develop with a 'full-blown depressive psychosis'.[1] In other cases the depressed person adopts the 'sick role', thereby reducing and modifying what is expected of him in life and increasing the amount of attention he will receive. Because loneliness and depression adversely affect a patient's attitude towards healing and rehabilitation, they may justly be described as causes of continuing illness.

There are several causes of isolation and possible consequent loneliness:

1. Bereavement.
2. Separation from adult children.
3. Retirement, with consequent loss of sense of achievement and usefulness.
4. Physical disability, which may cause loss of job, loss of social contacts, loss of self-sufficiency.

To these may be added the change in outlook seen in many of the ageing, a feeling of being out of date in a changing world, an inability to comprehend the outlook of others. There is often, in addition, a financial uncertainty or shortage which affects every activity of everyday life, leading to a narrowing of horizons.[2] All of these together can cause such a withdrawal from the community that, even when living with others in the communal home for the aged, the individual's isolation within himself persists and is frequently the precursor of psychiatric illness.

It has been said that loneliness may well be called the greatest problem of the aged.[3] What can music do to help?

Associations with the past may be evoked by several stimuli. Colours, scents, sounds—all these have the power to throw us back in time, and for a few moments we relive the events of the past. Sometimes our memories are pleasant, sometimes unpleasant, but all of us have at different times experienced the calling to mind of the past as a result of external stimuli.

Music shares these evocative powers, and fortunately the associations are usually pleasant. Our earliest memories, consciously or unconsciously, are often of a lullaby, and our memories of and responses to rhythmical stimuli may well be traced to pre-natal life, when the whole existence of the foetus is dominated by the maternal heartbeat. We may also have pleasant memories connected with songs of childhood, perhaps Sunday School hymns and choruses. And for many people there are, too, the special songs which bring memories of love and courtship. Even war songs may have happy associations, reminding us of the mateship of service life, and the recollection of being needed then by the community (a knowledge often lacking from the daily lives of so many people under ordinary circumstances).

It is this associative quality which gives to music its power to 'socialise'. Because elderly people tend to dwell in the past too much, it may seem unwise to accentuate this by calling up the past still more by music. The aim, however, should be to encourage discussion, relating one person's memories of a particular period of time with those of others in the group, to talk about the past in relation to the present (making this constructive in helping patients as far as possible to understand present-day attitudes rather than simply contributing the 'Aren't the younger generation awful!' type of conversation). In short, one should aim at intellectual stimulation, using reminiscence to build therapeutic discussion.

In social clubs for the elderly, music may play an important part in the activities which take place, in formal or informal ways. In some such clubs, singing is undertaken as a definite program of work, aiming at performance either for other members of the club, for similar clubs from other localities, or at a local musicale. Some members of clubs for the elderly may feel that the quality of their work does not lend itself to performance for others—especially when the music takes the form of singing, in which the ageing voice is at a definite disadvantage—and concentrate instead on the purely social aspects of music, with community singing as a regular feature of club activities. Serious study in musical appreciation and understanding may also be undertaken, following the syllabus or the general pattern of adult education classes. Such group activities have a secondary and often unrecognised benefit of teaching the aged to work in groups and expanding their range of social contacts by providing a different environment for the inter-action from that provided otherwise. As pointed out by Professor Adam Curle,[4] the new group member is in a situation he has never precisely experienced before, and new demands are made and new opportunities provided for the exploration of the personality. It may be felt that by the time people have reached the age described as 'elderly' such chances and demands are of little practical application, that most have their personalities already so firmly fixed that social interaction is not likely to be very productive. For some, this is undoubtedly so, but for others the full range of the personality may not have developed, and great satisfaction may be gained from new ways of developing human relationships—and music can provide such an environment.

At one time it was commonly believed that friendships were based on complementary principles, that 'opposites attract', but in recent years sociologists' research into the formation of friendships indicates that in fact relationships are more readily formed between persons who see themselves as having similar personality traits.[5] It does not seem to be stretching conclusions too far to infer that the sharing of strong common interests in a hobby or activity will, by emphasizing similarities in taste, foster the formation of new friendships.

Music provides such an avenue of shared interests and activities. These may be in simple community singing, in choral work in church or other choir, in adult education study group, or—at a more advanced level—in chamber music or amateur orchestra. Community singing, which demands no high level of performance, and in which even the 'growler' may be able to join unselfconsciously, is in some ways the most clearly therapeutic of these activities. An interesting description[6] has been given by a musically-minded social worker in London of the spontaneous singing of a group of people on a bus excursion, of the changes in mood of the songs which were sung. (In a more structured situation, the music therapist may deliberately manipulate the mood of the group by the songs which are sung, so long as this manipulation does not infringe the rights of the group to free choice.)

One of the problems which arise in those newly admitted to nursing homes or geriatric hospitals is the effect of the transfer, which may be either from their homes or from a hospital which can no longer cope with the patient's chronic condition. The

effects of the emotional trauma are seen in rapid deterioration
of the physical condition, and/or general emotional and psychological confusion and disturbance.

A medical social worker, Joseph Brudno, has suggested a program of pre-admission group therapy, whereby a number of
patients to be admitted at the same time meet for three sessions.[7]
The aim of these sessions is two-fold: to enable the patients to
discuss the possible effects of transfer before they happen, and thus
to mitigate these effects, and to establish the beginnings of new
social relationships with other patients/residents which will carry
them over the first period of readjustment. Brudno testifies to the
success of these measures.

In any hospital or rest home in which community musical
activities are a part of the program, it would be both feasible and
desirable to include some of these in such a pre-admission group
therapy plan. This would, in all probability, accentuate the beneficial group relationships established between patients in the
ready-to-admit group, and act as a preventive measure regarding
the initial isolation of transferred patients.

This is, in essence, the preventive intervention, anticipatory
guidance or emotional inoculation described by Gerald Caplan.[8]
The work he described was in connection with the American
Peace Corps; with children about to enter kindergarten; and with
pregnant women preparing for childbirth. But the principle—of
coping with the problem before it arises—is the same.

Can music justifiably be regarded as a branch of preventive
medicine? The answer one gives probably depends on the stress
one lays on psychogenic factors as a source of illness in the elderly.
Clearly a strong interest in some activity cannot prevent the
occurrence of a stroke. Macaulay, for example, one of the leading
intellectual figures of the nineteenth century, became a vapid
conversationalist as the result of a stroke sustained in his late
fifties. A strong interest can, however, prevent the elderly from
adopting the 'sick role' in life, with the depression which is such a
feature of this attitude. Furthermore, disuse disabilities and contractures are less likely to occur in a person who retains a vital
interest in a hobby than in one who just sits around all day. With
terminal cases, likewise, disuse syndromes are less likely to occur
when music is used in the ward, because it helps to maintain
alertness and spontaneous movements.

One is inevitably led on to discuss motivation in health and
sickness, and this will be discussed at greater length in a later

chapter. But one may sum up this section on socialisation by saying that all the evidence points to music as being for most people an easy and convenient way of encouraging social interaction, and a help in removing the barriers which so often divide one person from another.

REFERENCES

1. Sloane, R. and Frank, D. 'The mentally afflicted older person', *Journal of Geriatrics*, Nov. 1970, pp. 73-82.
2. Pritchard, H. M. 'Income requirements of the aged', in *The Aged in Australian Society*, (ed.) Sax, S., Angus and Robertson, Sydney, 1970, pp. 75-87.
3. Johnson, E. 'Social provision for the aged', in *Growing Old in the Australian Community*, (ed.) Stoller, A., Cheshire, Melbourne, 1960, pp. 46-53.
4. Curle, A. 'Group dynamics', in *Social Group Work*, (ed.) Kuenstler, P., Faber & Faber, London, 1955.
5. Izard, C. E. 'Personality similarity and friendships', in *Approaches, Contexts and Problems of Social Psychology*, (ed.) Sampson, E. E., Prentice-Hall, London, 1964, pp. 113-118.
6. Wilder, J. 'Music and the psychiatric rehabilitation association'; paper published by British Society for Music Therapy, 1964.
7. Brudno, J. 'Experimental approach to services for the ready-to-admit applicant to a geriatric home and hospital', *Journal of The American Geriatrics Society*, vol. XVI, no. 5, 1968, p. 597.
8. Caplan, G. *Principles of Preventive Psychiatry*, Tavistock, London, 1964, p. 94.

3. *Music in psychotherapy*

To what extent are the aged affected by mental illness? Should we think in terms of routine group work for those who do not need professional psychiatric care?

There are numerous problems of human relationships and the personality which trouble the elderly, but of these it seems likely that loneliness, grief and loss are the strongest. There are many causes of mental illness (and it has been estimated[1] that as many as eighty per cent of the elderly show mental symptoms, although only about eight per cent have a severe disability), but most of these conditions have their origins and first signs earlier in life, and they receive attention in later life only because it is at this stage that they become more noticeable.[2] Of the problems which are, in effect, the result of ageing, many can be helped by free discussion in a group setting, and music can be used to stimulate this. (Throughout this book 'psychotherapy' is not intended to imply psychoanalytical consultation, but general beneficial group work.)

What type of themes can be used as the centre of a musically-based discussion? The author has found that by careful choice of music, with planned 'leading questions', almost anything can be brought to the surface (see page 73 onwards).

Having brought out the thoughts which have caused anxieties and worry, what next? Does it in fact achieve anything, or is it merely upsetting people unnecessarily? The answer is that talking things over *does* help. One of the most frustrating things we can suffer is when people seem not to understand why we are unhappy, and believe that the things which trouble us are trivial and can be dealt with by saying, 'There, there, never mind, it will all come out in the wash', while we know that the worries will never be removed by such facile platitudes.

To discuss anxieties in a friendly atmosphere, in a group of people who either share some of the problems or who at least attempt to understand them, is in itself helpful and makes us feel that the troubles are easier to bear because we are not alone.

One of the most telling influences in the life of the elderly is grief, and its expression and the profound effects of inadequate expression have interested physicians.[3, 4, 5] It seems probable that repressed or inadequate grieving is responsible both for continuing depression and for the exacerbation of such conditions as rheumatoid arthritis.

Just as there are many causes for loneliness, so there are many causes for grief. The most obvious, grieving over the deaths of spouse, relatives and friends, is not the only source of distress for the elderly. One must consider the psychological effects of physical disability, whether this disability has come overnight (and 'overnight' is often a literal description of the onset of a stroke), or as an encroaching disability, such as Parkinson's disease. Some of those concerned with the habilitation and rehabilitation of the disabled go so far as to say that anyone with a physical disability, whether it is present from birth (as cerebral palsy or abnormal physical conformation) or acquired later in life (as, for example, a stroke), should be regarded as being at-risk from a psychological point of view. (The exceptions are those whose dependency needs are met by being ill, and who therefore do better when they are ill than when they are well.)

One must also consider the effects of separation from children. In this mobile age, separation because of business moves is common, taking from the aged the support which in earlier times was given by married children living nearby. The effects of retirement are another cause of grief, and one which sometimes receives inadequate attention. One may take the rather self-righteous attitude that people should prepare for their retirement in middle life, and not expect to adapt to a new way of life abruptly later. True, but most hobbies cost money, even if only for the purchase of fertilizers for the garden, and many elderly people cannot afford to keep up their hobbies on the reduced income available. Some men have the foresight to predict rising costs and equip themselves for retiring to their hobbies, purchasing such equipment as will be necessary while they are still earning sufficient income to do so. But many are overtaken almost unawares by rising costs.

One must understand the loss of a sense of achievement which is commonly experienced at retirement, a loss which few hobbies can outweigh. However much this loss is expected, it can never be comprehended until it is actually experienced. We all need to feel that the community needs us, and although some jobs give little satisfaction in this way, all of us have at times the happy experience of knowing that we are necessary cogs in the wheels of business, the community or other enterprise, even if our work consists of clearing the streets of rubbish. At retirement, our job satisfaction is gone, and the gold watch or engraved clock, however much they remind us of our days of usefulness, are no substitute. We must somehow give our retired people a new source of achievement, in community or other service.

Further causes of grief which have been discussed by those concerned with care of the elderly are the loss of senses, such as sight and hearing, and loss of self-sufficiency and consequent loss of dignity. In a most cogent article on loss,[6] which appeared in one of the journals published by the American Psychological Association, Burnside wrote of the recurrence of the theme in group work with the aged. She pointed out that bereavement as such is only one of the causes of grieving, another cause being the invalidism which eventually overtakes one partner in most long-term marriages, destroying the whole balance of the relationship—at worst making supportive the partner who has always been the dependent individual, or at best changing patterns of companionship and activity.

Loss of dignity is a topic which is not readily discussed, because it has connotations of grumbling, but when the confidence of the group has developed, one finds that this loss is a perpetual source of unhappiness—in particular when it springs from the loss of independence in coping with one's own bowel and bladder functions. Having to wait for a bedpan to be brought, the apparent callousness (and sometimes the actual callousness) of nurses who procrastinate in this matter, worrying over 'accidents' which may occur when there are long delays . . . these may be a source of great unhappiness to the patient because they remove from him his dignity as a person. Such worries may also lead to the patient becoming obsessed with these bodily functions, showing marked anxiety about them. The loss of people's attention is another source of indignity. The elderly in nursing homes often feel, and rightly so, that people do not listen to them, nurses often use baby-talk to them and give their opinions scant attention, even when these opinions are about new symptoms—which are not always as unfounded on fact as some nurses often profess to believe!

Security is threatened by loss of friends and familiar surroundings. The ageing frequently have to move to small apartments for the aged, giving up many of their treasures because of lack of space, or they may be in nursing homes where even such trivial personal possessions as photographs are discouraged or forbidden as making dusting more difficult. (Inhumane as this is, it does occur in some places.) This loss of familiar surroundings accentuates any mental confusion which exists, because the patient is disoriented by unfamiliarity.

One tends to think that in old age such problems as sex and marital relationships have sorted themselves out long ago, but this is not always so. The change in balance of relationships when one partner becomes entirely dependent upon the other has already been mentioned, and this is especially disruptive when the weaker partner has to become the supporting partner.

In retirement, lack of appropriate activity for the former breadwinner may cause marital disharmony because a man accustomed to business efficiency will often attempt to take over the running of a house, which the wife regards as her domain. She has previously reigned supreme, and resents the implication, stated or inferred, that she has been inefficient all the years before. She may, on the other hand, want a rest from household chores, and thus tries to involve her husband more closely than he wishes in the running of the home. Because of the diverse ages of parents when their children are born, it may not be until the later years of life that the last child leaves home, so that other difficulties may arise in feeling no longer needed by the family.

Yet another crisis which occasionally arises in old age is the necessity of placing a defective child in an institution because the aged parents can no longer care for him at home. This presents a doubly traumatic experience in that the parent feels guilty at no longer caring for the child and may also relive the original crisis when it was realised that the child was abnormal or subnormal, with all the disruptive effects on family life which the advent of such a child brings.

A marriage may also be placed under a strain in old age by the partners being together all the time. Many marriages which have appeared superficially successful in the middle years have really been so only because the partners have not spent a great deal of time together. The man has been engrossed in his work, often taking on extra work or long hours which have kept him away from home because, consciously or unconsciously, he has preferred to be away from home, and the wife has been utterly absorbed in domestic affairs. At retirement, however, they are together all the time, unless the husband has an absorbing hobby such as golf, and the fundamental lack of empathy between the partners comes to the surface for the first time. In some cases, it may even lead to complete breakdown of the marriage, and divorce, but more commonly it manifests itself in coldness and bickering, as well as exacerbating the effects of any disability which may develop in one or the other partner.

It will be seen that old age presents both crisis situations and long-term stress—the first in the initial reaction to death of loved ones, disability, change and loss, and the second in long-term loss of independence and dignity, prolonged invalidism or changes in patterns of married life.

Gerald Caplan in his outstanding book, *An Approach to Community Mental Health*, writes of the changing patterns of mourning, the lack of interpersonal communication and the way people are thrown more and more onto their own resources in dealing with crisis situations, and of the need for improvement of self in learning to deal with the crises of life. He also refers to the dangers of prescribing tranquillizers in crisis situations, pointing out that they damp down the healthy processes of adaptation in life problems.

In an article which originally appeared in the *American Journal of Psychiatry*, but which has since been reprinted in a book on crisis situations, Lindemann writes of 'grief work' as being the extricating of oneself from bondage to the deceased, and the finding of new patterns of rewarding interaction. He describes the abnormal patterns of grief (the denial, the morbid overreaction, and the distorted reaction which, instead of grief, presents changes in behaviour and other personal relationships). He states that when these abnormal patterns of grief are converted to normal by the working out of true grief work, then the patient can go on to live a normal life and embark on ordinary relationships.

Old age can present such a picture of sadness and disappointment that it may only seem surprising that more of the aged do not allow themselves to be overwhelmed by the narrowing of their horizons. Most of us can admit that our sorrows and disappointments are both real and justifiable, and we learn to live with them. As John Gardner writes in his stimulating book:[7]

Life is harsh, but it has always been harsh. The only sensible view of life is, and has always been, based on a clear-eyed recognition—not necessarily acceptance—of the elements of tragedy, irony and absurdity in life. It is based too on a recognition of one's own limitations and weaknesses, the inexorable facts of the life-cycle, and all the sorrow, irrationalities and indignities that affect the flesh and the spirit. Anyone who does not recognise all of this is either very young, or very foolish, possibly both.

Each of us seeks, in different ways at different times, 'conceptions of the universe that give dignity, purpose and sense to his own existence'.

However, some find it hard to accept such a realistic view of life, and even to themselves cannot admit their true feelings. All of us, to a greater or lesser degree, present a facade to the world and perhaps even to ourselves. Erving Goffman gives vivid illustrations of this,[8] describing the various roles we all play out in our relationships with others. 'Through social discipline, a mask of manner may be held in place from within.' Sometimes we become imprisoned in a mask of stoicism, and will not seek help from others, preferring to accept our troubles silently, or even denying that they exist. This attitude has become apparent in some of the surveys done in recent years, which have revealed many cases of illness which had never been reported to the medical practitioner. Sometimes failing vision, fading hearing, breathlessness, or 'getting up in the night' have been accepted because the person has seen them as the inescapable result of getting old,[9] even when in fact something could have been done about them. But sometimes it is clear, in talking with the aged, that they have all their lives scorned medicine as being for weaklings, and are too proud to let this stoical outlook go in old age. Such attitudes are hard to change.

Although few today would share Aristotle's views[10] on the power of music to change the soul, it is observed that music provides the right climate for what can be described as psychocatharsis, or, in more common language, 'getting things out of the system', and as far as possible, coming to terms with life in a realistic manner.

As pointed out previously, music has strong powers of association. In general, one uses these to build up a happy atmosphere, but, where normal grief work has never been developed, it is necessary to use music's associative powers to promote the working out of grief—the tears, fears, the guilt feelings. Sometimes one hears a patient criticized as being too tearful, and the unfortunate individual is either persistently jollied along or kept firmly in order without any inquiry as to whether there is a reason for tearfulness, and with no realization that to permit the full working out of grief might put an end to the tearfulness.

The difficulty in this is that for some hospital staff, even for those with a fairly objective view of their own personalities, signs of grieving in their patients set up an intolerable tension and anxiety, so that they feel that they must somehow stem the tears, rationalizing this by insisting that weeping is bad for the patient. At the other extreme is the person who welcomes the tears of others, not for their therapeutic benefit but for the opportunity afforded to pose as a comforter, offering not strength (as in the true meaning of comfort) but mere sentimental emotion. Ruthless self-analysis and willingness to control one's own reactions for the sake of others seem to offer the only solution to these problems, together with consultation with clinical psychologist or psychiatrist and with the rest of the therapeutic team.

When in the course of group discussion it becomes apparent that a patient has deeper psychological and emotional difficulties than can be dealt with in an informal and non-professional setting, what should be done? As Maddison asks in his article on crisis studies,[11] how can we decide what extent of abnormal or different behaviour justifies someone being regarded as a 'case'?

The answer varies from one culture to another, so that behaviour which in one culture would be regarded as psychotic may in another be regarded as normal or even desirable. (As, for example, the occurrence of trance in the traditional Balinese culture, and—in the same culture—much of the maternal rejection of children described in the pre-war study of Bali made by Margaret Mead and her colleague.[12])

And even in what is nominally a uniform, highly civilized culture, there are marked differences in attitude from one family to another, so that in one an eccentric grandparent may be a source of pride, but in another even mild symptoms of arteriosclerosis, such as vagueness and forgetfulness, result in such unbearable family tensions that the relative has to be cared for in a hospital or nursing home. Another point which may escape attention is that, while suffering from temporary stressful situations, people display apparent signs of mental illness which will subside spontaneously when the situations are put right, without any treatment being necessary.

In regard to specialist treatment in most medical or surgical specialties, there is seldom any difficulty in reaching a decision as to whether a referral is necessary, but when emotional and mental needs are at point, difficulties do often arise. Decision as to whether a patient in a geriatric unit should be referred for specialist treatment by a psychiatrist should be a matter for group inter-disciplinary discussion. The final decision will be influenced by several factors: the existence of stressful life situations which may cause temporary mental symptoms and whether these can be remedied; the availability of a clinical psychologist or psychiatrist who is interested in and sympathetic to the problems of old age; the attitude of the leader of the therapeutic team as to whether psychiatry is seen as offering hope for a happier way of life or as a punitive measure with which the patient is threatened if he fails to respond adequately to other forms of treatment. (Such an attitude is still observed.) Another factor may be the extent to which the team of therapists is organized as a therapeutic community, with free discussion on equal terms of all members (in which case the views of all will be taken into consideration) or as a benevolent autocracy in which decisions are made on a less co-operative basis.

Working without the support of a team, as for example in a small nursing home, one may have difficulty in deciding when to ask the patient's doctor for help in psychiatric problems. In his book on preventive psychiatry,[13] Caplan discusses the vital need for early referral in psychiatric illness, so that unhealthy patterns of behaviour in coping with crises do not become a settled part of the patient's life. He suggests that there should be leaflets available giving not only the symptoms which should alert us to mental illness but also a list of facilities available, such as walk-in clinics comparable with casualty departments in general hospitals. He points out that some people do better under treatment when certain euphemisms are employed to refer to their illness, so that they think of themselves as seeking help in solving personal problems rather than thinking of themselves as being mentally ill. The stigma of mental illness is such that even hospital staff often hesitate to refer patients for psychiatric consultation, but the realization that early referral may prevent much long-term disability should deter us from such hesitation. Obvious signs which indicate that treatment is necessary are such observations as delusions (e.g. that food is poisoned or that the patient has ceased to exist as a person), hallucinations, either auditory or visual, and great feelings of guilt, which accompany acute depression. These are so clear that few of us would hesitate to ask for professional specialist help for patients under these conditions, but when symptoms are less obvious, decisions may be harder. Encouraging patients to talk things over in music session may help to make a decision clearer, showing whether the patient is coping rationally with whatever the problem is, or whether he is adopting magical thinking or other unrealistic ways of dealing with life situations.

The opportunities for using music in individual therapy depend on the staff available. In America, referral for individual treatment by music therapists is fairly common, although this seems to be for behaviour problems in younger subjects and for frank psychiatric cases. But, given appropriate resources, individual work in music with the elderly is very helpful, especially in stimulating interest in music as a hobby.

One case in which this was most effective was that of a man, aphasic as the result of a stroke, who had had an interest in music in earlier life. Individual sessions were arranged, these taking the form of studying the published radio program. Pencil marks were placed beside items in which the patient showed interest. Programs for the previous week were also studied, the patient having marked those items which he had heard at home, and indicating by facial expression whether or not he had enjoyed them. Gradually his renewed interest in music gave him greater powers of concentration in general (as described by his wife) and his interests in television also changed. After his stroke, but before the music sessions were started, the patient's wife had been worried by his obsessive interest in violence as seen in TV programs, but, as his interest in music increased, this obsession faded. Fortunately, the family's financial position was such that they were able to buy tape recording apparatus, so that the patient's interest in music developed in a constructive way. His interest has persisted over a considerable period of time. This is not the only form of individual work which might be undertaken. Each person who undertakes therapeutic work can develop his own ideas, according to his own preferences and abilities.

A question was posed at the beginning of this chapter about the general need for group work. The answer is plain. From the writings of those who work with the aged, it is clear that the difficulties of adjusting to disability are such that everyone in a rehabilitation unit will have something they need to talk about in a supportive atmosphere with others who have similar problems.[14] Although it is possible to organize such a group without any external 'trigger', the task is easier when music provides relaxation and warmth of atmosphere. It is to be hoped that all rehabilitation units, whether purpose-built or not, will have provision made for therapeutic group work.

REFERENCES

1. Kay, D., Beamish, P. and Roth, M. 'Old age mental disorders in Newcastle-upon-Tyne', *British Journal of Psychiatry*, 1964, vol. 110, pp. 146-158.
2. Sloane, R. and Frank, D. 'The mentally afflicted older person', *Journal of Geriatrics*, Nov. 1970, pp. 73-82.
3. Caplan, G. *An Approach to Community Mental Health*, Tavistock, London, 1961, pp. 58-63, 219-222, 224-5.
4. Lindemann, E. 'Symptomatology and management of acute grief', *American Journal of Psychiatry*, 1944, vol. 101, p. 141.
5. Gramlich, E. 'Recognition and management of grief in elderly patients', *Geriatrics*, July 1969, pp. 87-92.
6. Burnside, I. M. 'Loss—a constant theme in work with the aged', *Hospital and Community Psychiatry*, 1970, vol. 21, no. 6, pp. 173-7.
7. Gardner, J. *Self-Renewal*, Harper, New York, 1965, p. 111.
8. Goffman, E. *The Presentation of Self in Everyday Life*, Doubleday/Anchor, New York, 1959, p. 57.
9. Andrews, G. 'Preventive geriatrics: is it possible?', *Journal of Geriatrics*, Nov. 1970, p. 26.
10. Aristotle, *Politics*, Book VIII, 5-7.
11. Maddison, D. 'Epidemiology and after: the implications of crisis studies', in *Psychiatry and The Community*, (eds.) Maddison, D. and Pilowsky, I., Sydney University Press, 1969, pp. 51-63.
12. Mead, M. and Bateson, G., *Balinese Character*, Academy of Science, New York, 1962.
13. Caplan, G. *Principles of Preventive Psychiatry*, Tavistock, London, 1964.
14. Hirschberg, G., Lewis, L. and Thomas, D. *Rehabilitation*, Lippincott, Philadelphia, 1964, p. 62.

4. *Music in psychotherapy—the group*

In the previous chapter, there was a tacit assumption that the group exists as a therapeutic entity, and it is appropriate that there should be included here a brief discussion as to whether this is so, and of some of the ideas about group relationships which have been formulated in the twentieth century.

One of the controversies in group dynamics is whether there should be separate theories on dynamics and general social inter-action in each type of group, or whether there should be general theories only, applicable to all, with variations for each type of group.[1] The disadvantage of the first system is that the number of different types of groups is almost unlimited. One sees, for example, such contrasting bodies as a gang of juvenile delinquents, three churchwardens, the shareholders of a vast industrial enter-prise, a small two-generation family, a trade union, a cricket team, an adult education discussion group, and a brownie-guide 'six'. Thus the number of separate theories which becomes necessary is likewise almost innumerable. But on the other hand, if one propounds only general theories, there is a danger that they will by necessity be so general in their terms of reference that they will not say very much.

There are many points of interest to the general reader in studies of group dynamics, since all of us belong consciously or unconsciously to several groups in our lifetime, many of them simultaneously. Topics which one finds discussed in books on group theory are, for example, concerned with the cohesiveness of groups, the way a group chooses a leader, the effects of indi-vidual personalities on the life and achievements of a group, and the establishment of norms within the group's behaviour and attitudes. One of the most controversial matters, which arose first in the 1920s but is still discussed, is concerned with the ques-tion of whether there is a group personality as such which is different from the sum total of personalities of the individual members, or whether there can be no other personality than that given to the group by its separate participants.[2] The two names most closely associated with this controversy were those of William McDougall and Floyd Allport, the first maintaining the reality of a composite group character, the other the sole reality of the individual personality.

In discussion about groups, division is often in terms of primary and secondary groups, 'primary' being those in which numbers are fairly small and in which there is face-to-face contact, and 'secondary' those in which numbers are large, members being held together by common ideals or themes, but with little face-to-face contact.[3] A family provides a clear example of a primary group, while a trade union demonstrates a secondary group (although in any given work situation or factory, there will be sub-groups of the union, in which members are held together by the same ideals etc. as the parent body, but who in themselves form a primary group as well). Division of groups may also be on the basis of permanency or impermanency.

A long-stay hospital or nursing home may constitute a permanent primary group, altered only by death, but primary groups may also be temporary, as is seen *par excellence* in a holiday fraternity formed on board ship òr at a resort. Although lasting group relationships are sometimes formed under these circumstances, these are exceptional. Most of us have had the experience of meeting, under everyday conditions, those whom on holiday we have regarded as friends, and wondering what we had ever had in common.

Until fairly recently, what has been called 'the doctrine of work' made people feel that they should form groups only in order to improve themselves physically, spiritually or mentally. Nowadays, however, we recognize the provision of companionship as sufficient justification alone for the formation of groups, and so we see the setting up of social clubs for young and old. (On the whole, those in middle life are usually too busy with family life for social clubs only, and tend to belong to a purpose-oriented body, either for sport, or a service organization such as Rotary, or a hobby group such as a choir, or else to a religious-centred group connected with church or synagogue.)

For the young, many social clubs have the unexpressed aim of finding a mate, and when this has been achieved membership changes to one of the organizations listed above. But for the el-

c

derly, social groups are of a more lasting nature, and although individual membership sometimes lapses because of friction between members, more often it lasts until broken by death or until severe disabling illness intervenes. Such group relationships can have a very real therapeutic value.

In therapeutic work in hospital, nursing home or other geriatric group, one tries to build up an atmosphere of optimism, freedom of thought and support between individuals, and it is in this context that the controversy referred to earlier regarding group personality is relevant to the present discussion. If there can be a group personality, which can, as has been suggested, survive even a total change of membership, then our task will be the easier, because once the required atmosphere has been established, new patients and new staff will be drawn into it, with beneficial results. If, however, no such group personality can be established, then the climate of thought and feeling must be re-established with each change of personnel. What really happens, as far as we can tell from observing geriatric rehabilitation or care?

It is possible that in this context, at least, there need be no dichotomy between the two schools of thought. Each of us has different traits of character, often even conflicting traits, which are brought to the surface in different circumstances. For example, each of us may on some occasions appear brave, on others timid, sometimes hopeful and sometimes despondent. Expectations of what any group offers, its reputation and its avowed purpose, may bring to the surface traits which are not otherwise necessarily the *dominant* traits of each individual, but which are nevertheless true parts of the personality of each. Thus people attending a unit which is established to provide rehabilitation and which is staffed by experts in this field have their rose-coloured spectacles on, and their traits of optimism are seen, even if—in general—they are not very noticeably optimistic people. In this way a group climate of hope is set up, which, so long as there is not a wholesale change of staff and patients simultaneously, should survive changes in personnel. And even in this eventuality, the unit's reputation alone may be enough to provide continuity of atmosphere.

We are seeing apparently the growth of a group personality as such, but what we are really seeing is the simultaneous development of such beneficial traits as hope, tolerance and perseverance, and the diminution or extinction of such traits as despair, intolerance and impatience in each individual. Free discussion, in a musical milieu, can help the establishment of such an atmosphere.

So far, examples have been drawn from the field of therapy, but it is interesting to see also the effects of mass morale or atmosphere in other circumstances. Accounts of mass emotion, usually at variance with normal behaviour, are found throughout history. One interesting example, from a musical point of view, is found in accounts of outbreaks of tarantism, characterized by extraordinary mass dancing with epileptiform seizures.[4] These were said to be the result of bites of the tarantula spider, but were probably hysterical in origin. The outbreaks were still seen in Italy in the nineteenth century, and those affected were said to be cured by the playing of suitable music, fiddlers being employed to be ready to play when necessary in the harvest fields. The *Oxford Companion to Music* refers to the difference in the types of music which were alleged to cure the condition, and comments, 'Presumably it does not matter what music is used provided one perspires freely in a mood of faith'. But in this, as in those examples which follow, the *mass* character may still only be accounted for by the total traits of the members, even though these traits may not always appear on the surface.

Of greater significance in our own time was the mass enthusiasm and mass hysteria engendered at rallies of the Third Reich when addressed by Adolf Hitler. In Germany at that time, the identification of the individual with the aims of the Nazi party was almost complete, and there developed a long-lasting group personality devoted to the building up of the Aryan race and the ousting of all non-conformists, whether their non-conformism was a matter or race, religion or attitude.

At the same period of history, beneficial effects of high group morale were seen in England. It had been expected that prolonged bombing would cause widespread and severe incidence of mental illness, but this did not happen. Fortunately, the generally high morale of the English civilian proved to be very supportive, and little neurosis or psychosis was reported apart from bed-wetting among children who were taken from cities to the country to escape air-raids.[5] The singing of patriotic songs in the air-raid shelters helped to maintain a cheerful atmosphere despite the stressful situation.

It can be seen, then, that conformity to a 'group personality' can take precedence over individual traits, for good or ill. Erich Fromm writes of the bad effects of conformity, the loss of free will and of the conscience and thought of the individual in the development of the group.[6] Although his book is coloured by the times in which it was written (it was published in 1942), it has nevertheless a truth for all time, for hospital community or social club as for political party. We must beware lest, despite our therapeutic aim, we lay such stress on the value of group work that the non-conformist is made to feel ill at ease or even guilty. We must never allow ourselves to become what might be described as 'stifled by mateship'. Each of us needs to feel 'special'[7] sometimes.

Pressure to conform to the group has been used for therapeutic ends by such bodies as Alcoholics Anonymous and the various anti-obesity clubs which have been formed in many parts of the world. Here the willpower of the individual is reinforced by the desire to conform to the aims of the group, and by fear of possible 'punishment' in the disapproval of the group (even though such disapproval may not officially exist) in cases of backsliding.

In the weight-watching clubs, little cognizance seems to be taken of the reasons for obesity, but beneficial results are seen (although one wonders what serious long-term follow-up studies would reveal). This technique, of conformity and fear of disapproval, may be seen as a triumph for behaviourist philosophy, in treating the symptoms rather than the cause, but the group setting is undoubtedly an essential factor in the achievement of the aim of these activities.

In physical rehabilitation, group work, too, has a place. As long ago as 1924 it was found that the presence of a small audience brought improved performance in physical tasks and co-ordination.[8] Obviously we need onlookers to encourage us to do our best. This has undoubted therapeutic applications. Even in the treatment of such an 'individual' lesion as a stroke, in which no two cases are identical, evidence indicates that group rehabilitation is more successful than individual work.

In a study described by Dr S. Kurasik,[9] two groups of patients were treated, the one in a group as such, and the other as a control group in which patients were dealt with individually. At the end of eight weeks, there was a significant difference between the two groups, those who had been treated *en masse* showing markedly greater improvement than those who had received only individual attention. Dr Kurasik's conclusions were that in a group the patient sees himself as one of a number of fellow patients who share his worries, his physical problems and his needs. He can also envisage how he will adapt to his handicaps and compete with others who have similar disabilities.

In many day hospitals/wards/centres, patients are treated simultaneously, although not in a group as such. Patients under these conditions do observe the progress of others, compare notes at lunchtime as to progress, and are generally supportive to each other. Although not precisely under the conditions described by Dr Kurasik, the results are comparable with those he showed. In some day units, patients take part in group exercises as well as individual treatment, with further physical and psychological benefit.

In general keep-fit work, reports from the Camden Clinic in London[10] and from the Sonnestraal Geriatric Hospital in Hilversum, Holland indicate the value of group exercises. (It may seem surprising that general physical training should be necessary in addition to physiotherapy for symptoms of disability, but there is often a lessening of general stamina, apart from the disability as such, which can be assisted.) It is felt that group physical training, often performed to music, builds up good morale as well as a high level of physical fitness. Professor Schreuder of Hilversum describes how 'doubting Thomases' from the medical profession are invited to join in the physical training but generally drop out, exhausted, long before the elderly patients have given up![11]

In problem solving, several workers have tried to assess the effectiveness of the group as compared with the individual in solving problems. As Sprott[3] sums it up, 'Are two heads better than one? How many cooks spoil the broth?' Opinion is that, given adequate motivation, groups are better at problem-solving than individuals are. Perhaps rehabilitation is not exactly a problem to be solved, but for each individual patient and for each member of staff there are continual problems to be solved, continual challenges to be met, and the support of the group, whether patients, staff or both, may produce new ideas and new concepts—and new courage in facing the future.

We may summarize the intrinsic possibilities of group work in the words of John Cohen:

Provided members feel free to utter their thoughts, and provided they listen, the group in which they participate offers opportunities of assimilating the ideas of others and of accommodating to them which are perhaps otherwise unattainable.[12]

To sum up the value of music in providing an informal setting in group relationships and 'grass-roots psychotherapy', it seems relevant to quote again from Prof. Curle's article on group dynamics.[13] He is writing of the success of early work done in the days before theory and practice had become sophisticated, with therapy carried out, as it were, blindfold—'This leads one to suspect that there is something intrinsic in the group situation which is of value to the personality, and that the activity of the psychiatrist, or whoever happens to be in charge, is of almost secondary importance. He can, of course, disrupt the group atmosphere, but it seems likely that his success depends no less upon any positive contribution he may make than upon his ability to maintain an atmosphere in which the group can work upon itself.'

This, then, is the justification for such work based on music as has been described: it provides a suitable atmosphere in which the group concerned can work upon itself.

REFERENCES

1. Cartwright, D. and Zander, A. *Group Dynamics, Research and Theory*, Harper and Row, New York, 1968, p. 57.
2. *Ibid.* pp. 24ff.
3. Sprott, W. J. H. *Human Groups*, Penguin Books, Harmondsworth, 1958, p. 16 and p. 111.
4. Scholes, P. *Oxford Companion to Music*, Oxford University Press, 1947: Entry on Tarantism.
5. Norton, A. *The New Dimensions of Medicine*, Hodder and Stoughton, London, 1969, p. 130.
6. Fromm, E. *Fear of Freedom*, Routledge and Kegan Paul, London, 1942.
7. Stanton, A. H. and Schwartz, M. S. *The Mental Hospital*, Basic Books, New York, 1954, p. 300.
8. Travis, L. E. 'The effect of a small audience upon eye-hand co-ordination', *Journal of Abnormal and Social Psychology*, July 1925, pp. 142-6.
9. Kurasik, S. 'Group dynamics in rehabilitation of hemiplaegic patients', *Journal of The American Geriatrics Society*, vol. XV, no. 19, 1967, pp. 852-5.
10. Somerville, J. (Camden Road Rehabilitation Clinic), *personal communication*.
11. Schreuder, J. Th. 'Maintaining physical fitness as a therapeutic measure in old age', *Triangle 8*, 1968, p. 329 and *personal communication*.
12. Cohen, J. 'Contact between minds', in *Readings in Psychology* (ed.) Cohen, J., Allen and Unwin, London, 1964, p. 249.
13. Curle, A. 'Group dynamics', in *Social Group Work*, (ed.) Kuenstler, P., Faber and Faber, 1955, p. 142.

5. *Motivation and achievement*

Motivation may be described as one of the great 'why's' of human existence, and as such it must concern all those who work with the sick or ageing. It is the subject of much speculation and many words, and conferences on the topic are held in different parts of the world each year. Clearly, then, it is not feasible here to go into detailed theories of motivation, but some discussion is helpful in enabling us to understand the underlying feelings and needs of patients and in making some of the apparent paradoxes of behaviour more comprehensible.

At one time it was thought that behaviour was motivated only by the satisfying of the basic biological requirements of food, survival and reproduction of the species. However, it became obvious that, even at its simplest, human behaviour is far more complex than this, and that even in the other primates there are needs such as curiosity and problem-solving which must be met to provide a satisfying existence.

The two main schools of thought on motivation are those based on homeostasis and on hedonism.[1] Homeostasis comes from the Greek words 'homoiio' meaning 'like' and 'stasis' meaning 'standing'. (Homoiio is not to be confused with the similar Greek word 'homo', meaning 'the same' or 'identical'.) Followers of this school believe that there is a force within us which tends towards the maintaining of a similar status in our existence, or, as it is sometimes expressed, towards the reduction of tension. Applied to hunger, for example, this means that we eat in order to restore the status quo, reducing the tension produced in us by hunger. Hedonism, from the Greek word for pleasure, takes cognizance of our need for enjoyment of life, and believes that the need for happiness is the driving force behind our actions.

From the therapist's point of view these theories may or may not be interesting, and their application to therapeutic techniques may seem but slight, unless we equate 'motivation' with 'wanting' and 'drive'.

Probably the most interesting question concerned with motivation in hospital work is, 'Why do some people get better, and others, who have no apparent cause for *not* improving, not get better?' As Balint's study underlines, the cause may lie in the doctor himself.[2] The most potent drug in the whole pharmacopoeia—and the one about which least is known—is the drug 'doctor'. Although the study described in Balint's book was concerned with relationships in general practice, many of the conclusions do apply to any therapeutic relationship, since the degree of empathy between patient and therapist is crucial to the ultimate success or failure of any rehabilitative work. This is seen in every unit occasionally, when a patient who has been described as 'hopeless' suddenly improves when there is a change of staff, and at the same time a patient who has been doing well ceases to do so—as the result of the same change.

Some patients apparently do not want to get better. The reasons for this are various, and often hard to uncover. However, in discussion groups based on music, patients do often reveal attitudes towards their disability, towards rehabilitation and towards their families which otherwise remain hidden. Some patients talk about these quite openly, others reveal their inner attitudes only in the phenomenon of projection. (This is one of the defence mechanisms of the personality, in which traits which are unacceptable and cannot even be acknowledged in the conscious thoughts are ascribed to other things or other people. A good example of this is seen in the way our own irritating characteristics, which we often fail to recognise in ourselves, tend to annoy us when we see them in others, and indeed we may even ascribe these traits to people who in fact do not exhibit them at all.) Projection tests are the basis of many techniques for psychological testing, varying from the Rorschach ink-blot tests to the more structured Murray Thematic Apperception Tests.

Music, by relaxing and by stimulating free association of ideas, tends towards the revelation of inner, hidden attitudes, through this phenomenon of projection. The motives which may be revealed for 'not getting better' are often one of the following:

1. The patient may be one whose dependency needs have never been met, who enjoys either the extra attention which illness bestows, or the reduced expectations from family and community, and the general aura which illness confers. Some patients who

say they wish to be helped by attending, for example, a day hospital, may in fact be seeking the status of patient for its own sake. (Chronic depression is commonly seen in this syndrome.)

2. The patient, usually a younger man, may fear the effects of disability on his earning power and on his position on the status ladder of the community. Such patients put off getting better because they are unwilling to face the possibility of a change in their way of life.

3. Others, and these are the easiest to understand, have simply lost heart, either because of the intractable nature of their disability, or because what Professor Wylie has called 'the emotional erosion of long disability' has weakened their desire to recover.[3] Clearly, the invariable referral of stroke patients in the first stages of their condition would obviate this last cause for lack of motivation.

Patients who fit into the first of the descriptions above are not easy to spot at the initial assessment, and, if undetected, are a source of worry and irritation to the therapist, who feels frustrated that her efforts meet with no success and is puzzled as to why this should be so. However, this negative motivation in the patient may well be uncovered in musical work, and—once the problem is uncovered and reported to the rest of the clinical team —steps may be instituted to deal with it.

Professor Henry Mark, director of a department of behavioural science in Baltimore, wrote in the journal *Geriatrics* of the need for problem-solving for the elderly.[4] Dr Mark, who described himself as a hedonist in his beliefs on motivation, said that merely learning to live with a disability and the learning of new skills to compensate for loss of motor skills do not provide enough interest in life, and that people need to use their minds in an intellectual way too. (One wonders whether the present rather pragmatic approach to rehabilitation is at fault here, in that we spend time mainly on those pursuits which have an obvious use in daily living and almost ignore the intellectual and aesthetic needs of the patient. The author hopes that musical activities help to counterbalance such tendencies.)

Dr Mark suggests that even for those permanently in nursing homes or hospitals we may provide opportunities for problem-solving by encouraging the patients to run their own wards, to arrange their own programs of activity and to sort out personal difficulties which arise. (In the occupational therapy activities which were carried out in Australian Army medical work in the

1940s, this was done with good results.[5]) However, Dr Mark pointed out that to embark on a general 'use your mind' campaign for the elderly in the community might not be doing them any kindness, unless the community can be persuaded to alter its attitudes towards the potential contribution of the elderly, and to make use of the skills which would be resurrected by such a campaign. He said that the dulling of the intellect may be a merciful way of enabling the ageing to live with dignity in a world which offers them reduced achievements and usefulness. Truly an indictment of our society today.

The organizing of record programs and singing sessions can provide, on a small scale, a suitable opportunity for problem-solving by patients.

Motivation towards healing may be stimulated by the presence of others, not only because their presence 'puts us on our mettle', but also because 'group therapy with the aged may improve motivation by encouraging inter-personal relationships, and by providing instances of other similarly disabled patients making progress towards independence'.[6]

This leads on naturally to a discussion of achievement, and the spiral effect which is seen. Starting with some motivation towards rehabilitation, this is usually followed by some degree of success in rehabilitative work. This engenders further enthusiasm, which in turn makes it likely that there will be more success, and so on. Since a considerable amount of spontaneous improvement occurs in most cases of stroke, the morale of the group is usually high, and this again engenders stronger motivation towards regaining independence. Not all rehabilitative work in a geriatric unit is, of course, devoted to the treatment of cerebrovascular accidents. But even in the degenerative diseases such as Parkinsonism and multiple sclerosis, or in vascular or respiratory conditions, so much can be done to help the patient to make the most of what he has that morale can generally be sustained.

Some cases in which music played a significant role in improving motivation:

1. The patient was suffering from a severe steroid myopathy, acquired as the result of treatment with massive doses of prednisone to check an outbreak of pemphigus vulgaris. He had become very depressed and had lost interest in life to such an extent that it seemed likely that he would have to be sent to a long-term psychiatric ward. However, he was encouraged to enter a music group and started to join in the singing, choosing

his favourite songs and talking about them. His depression began to lift, and he began to use percussion instruments with built-up handles to join in informal band work. He also developed leg muscles working with a musical accompaniment on a bicycle device. Although music cannot be claimed to have effected a cure, it was felt that the patient's motivation was significantly improved by participation in musical group work.

2. The patient was suffering from multiple sclerosis, with considerable involvement of breathing and speech. She did not exhibit the characteristic euphoria of the disease, but was often very unhappy and tired very easily. She was willing to try to join in group singing, and, with the help of the speech therapist and physiotherapist, her control over her breathing was improved and she gained great satisfaction in her singing, especially when a tape-recording was played back to her. Music helped to give her a sense of achievement and the satisfaction of joining in an activity with others. Her ability to sing with the correct pitch was surprising, and in general the articulation was better in singing than in speech. (This has also been observed in advanced cases of Parkinsonism.) This patient's motivation in her work appeared to derive benefit from the activities in music.

In psychogeriatric work, music provides an excellent encouragement in motivation, helping the patients not only to maintain or regain an interest in life, counteracting to some extent that withdrawal into apathy which was at one time given the name of 'the institutional neurosis', but also providing motivation in physical work. Psychogeriatric patients with physical disabilities are hard to rehabilitate because they are, in general, not interested. Nevertheless, it is not uncommon to see a patient, thought to be virtually chair-bound despite the best efforts of nursing staff, get up and waltz around the room when music which 'takes the fancy' is played. For others, restorative exercises (which are resisted when presented as rehabilitation *per se*) are performed enthusiastically when presented as a game or an action song. Patients who have had a prosthesis inserted for the treatment of a broken femur are often apprehensive about weight-bearing, but by a combined effort of nursing staff to give initial support, and the music therapist to play appropriate music, it has been possible on several occasions to get these patients onto their feet again. In such cases, the physiotherapist makes suggestions as to what type and duration of movements should be undertaken. One patient had severe burns which had left adhesions under the arm which severely inhibited the upward movements of the arm. Since the patient was aphasic and virtually beyond communication, the efforts of physiotherapists to deal with these adhesions had not been successful. However, the patient was very interested in music, and by encouraging him to use instruments which involve upward movements of the arms, he attained a greater degree of freedom in movements of the limb.

Many other examples could be given of music as a motivating force in hospital work, but it is hoped that those outlined here will demonstrate some of its potential for helping those whose interest in attaining independence has become impaired.

Mention must be made of experimental work in motivation concerning persistence at a task as related to expectations of success and achievement motivation.[7] It was found that subjects showed greater persistence when they believed that their efforts would be successful than when they were motivated only by fear of failure. The implications of this in medical work are clear, and of vital importance in our presentation of therapy. Patients who believe that their work is going to be successful, as the result of the way it was presented to them by the therapist, are more likely to keep at it than those to whom the main emphasis was placed on the unpleasant consequences of *not* working hard.

REFERENCES

1. Mace, C. A. 'Homeostasis, needs and values', in *Readings in Psychology* (ed.) Cohen, J., Allen and Unwin, London, 1964, pp. 104-121.
2. Balint, M. *The Doctor, His Patient and The Illness,* (2nd edn.) Pitman Medical, London, 1964.
3. Wylie, C. M. (Dept. of Community Health, University of Michigan, U.S.A.), *personal communication.*
4. Mark, H. S. 'Mental challenge essential to the aged for "the good life"' *Geriatrics,* vol. 25, no. 5, pp. 41-50.
5. Walters, M. (Occupational Therapist), *personal communication.*
6. Hyams, D. E. 'Psychological factors in rehabilitation of the elderly', *Gerontologia Clinica,* vol. 11, March 1969, pp. 129-136.
7. Feather, N. T. 'Relating of persistence at a task to success and achievement—related motivation', in *Approaches, Contexts and Problems of Social Psychology,* Prentice-Hall, London, 1964, pp. 141-152.

6. *Music and learning*

What is learning, as applied to rehabilitation, and how can music be applied to the processes of learning in a therapeutic setting? Learning has been described as a change in behaviour which results from practice, and also as the cumulative effect of past behaviour on present behaviour.[1] For learning to take place, there must be a reward, or reinforcement, which results from successful completion of whatever task is being learned, and which makes it 'stick in our minds'. This reward may be a tangible one, as when animals being trained are rewarded with food, or it may be an intangible one, such as a sense of satisfaction.

Writers on learning make a distinction between classical conditioning, in which there is only one response (as, for example, in Pavlov's famous experiments in which he trained dogs to salivate at the sound of a bell or a metronome), and the trial-and-error type of learning, in which the subject tries a number of responses, being rewarded when the correct solution is eventually performed (e.g. a rat running a complex maze).

Learning involves both physiological and psychological factors, and the processes cannot be fully understood unless one recognizes that this is so. In order that learning should take place, there must be a drive, the motivation discussed in the previous chapter, and there must also be good teaching technique which takes into account all the processes by which information is transmitted to the brain, stored and retrieved.

Although some aspects of therapy and general treatment do not entail any learning, much of the treatment of disability does involve the learning processes, either in acquiring new techniques of daily living, or new techniques of physical activity such as walking after hemiplaegia, or in the learning of exercises which will assist in physical therapy.

With some exceptions (those who cannot understand what is

required of them because of a receptive aphasia; those who because of a parietal lesion are unaware of the affected parts of
the body; or those who for psychological reasons do not want to
be rehabilitated), the wish to learn presents no difficulty. Patients
want to get better and are willing to submit to discomfort or
inconvenience in order to do so.

The critical factors on which success in rehabilitation depends
are therefore: The patient's disability and how far it admits of
improvement; the learning/teaching techniques used in presenting aspects of therapy; the remembering of the exercises and
adaptations to living with a disability which have been taught.

Memory in the aged does present problems. Some research done
in Sweden by Dr Holger Hyden suggests that faulty memory is
due to breakdown in the formation of proteins in areas of the
brain, and later work has localized this area as being in the hippo-
campus.[2] Other research work has indicated that in the aged the
fault may lie in initial perception and retrieval as well as in the
storage of information.[3, 4] It is also true that good health is necessary for good memory.

In the matter of retrieval, there does not seem to be a great
deal we can do, except to ensure that a calm emotional atmosphere is maintained to lessen the occurrence of that type of forgetting which most of us know—namely, the 'mental block' which
makes us unable to remember things when under stress. Thus, in
learning to walk again, after stroke or fractured femur, music
assists the memory by relaxing tension and giving correct rhythm.

Regarding the initial perception of material, our teaching
methods are factors which an influence this. (Something which
has not been well understood in the first place is not likely to be
well remembered later.) In this we are hampered, of course, by
the receptive aphasia which is a common feature of a stroke
affecting the dominant hemisphere. Probably many patients who
appear obstinate have in fact never fully understood what was
required of them.

In a geriatric unit we see two main types of learning:

• the re-learning of motor skills which have been lost or impaired as the result of injury or illness; and

• the learning of new skills to compensate for skills which have
  been permanently lost or impaired. For example, a patient
  who is partly paralysed as the result of a stroke will 1. if
  possible learn to use again the paralysed parts of the body,

and 2. learn new methods—e.g. of dressing and walking—to compensate for the loss which remains despite the relearning.

As has already been mentioned, one of the problems of teaching the aged is their forgetfulness, and one must be prepared for this, and be willing to go over the lessons step by step as if for the first time. It is worthwhile considering the use of musical accompaniment to some work, to build up a sense of rhythm, and to jog the memory in regard to the nature of the work to be performed (e.g. in diaphragmatic exercises for emphysema.) This can be done only in large units, where there is space enough to organize remedial gymnastics with a musical accompaniment without disturbing the work of other therapists.

It is worth remarking here that psychologists have found that meaningful material is learnt better than meaningless material. The implications for the therapists are clear: one must show the purpose of work done, and not think it will be enough to say, 'This will be good for you'.

Rhythm and relaxation as assets to therapeutic work are seen in other work besides the treatment of hemiplaegia. For many disabled patients, breathing methods deteriorate, so that only the apex of the lungs is being used, with foreseeable consequences. Breathing exercises done to music should help to improve the patient's ventilation, within the limits imposed by the fundamental structure or defects of the lungs. The musical accompaniment gives a sense of rhythm, and helps the patient to learn the new techniques more easily. For those whose breathing is severely affected, as, for example, in multiple sclerosis, there may be an additional hazard of fear, and to induce relaxation by musical means will again improve the patient's learning of new methods and of making the most of the muscular resources which remain.

One of the senses which is sometimes lost after brain damage is the sense of position, and music can be used here to rebuild a patient's sensations of personal and extra-personal space. By using a musical instrument which produces a sound as soon as it is moved (such as sleighbells which jingle very easily), one can increase the patient's awareness of the position in space of hand or arm, since any movement produces an audible signal to the brain which can be perceived as indicating where the arm is placed. Such techniques are confined to the upper limbs, because the use of sleigh bells on the feet would seem ludicrous, reminiscent of the nursery rhyme 'Banbury Cross'! By encouraging the patient to watch the arm as well as listening to the sound, one builds up awareness of space by a two-fold sensory stimulus.

For patients who (because of damage to the parietal lobe of the brain) have lost track of where the parts of the body are, other musical techniques can be used. This is seen for example in Gerstmann's syndrome, in which there is an inability to distinguish one finger from the other when the fingers are interlaced, and an inability to know which hand the fingers belong to. Other patients demonstrate an inability to tell left from right, (somatolateral agnosia) and for them, too, music can help in the rebuilding of the lost senses. In both of these conditions, songs are used which name parts of the body at the same time as they are touched by the patient, so that learning takes place by a dual pathway, through tactile sensation in the touching of parts of the body and by audible stimulus in the rhythm and tune of the song.

This leads on to the problem of transfer of training, since it would be useless if the patient had to sing right through a song in order to decide where his nose was! A technique which has proved successful is:

1. At first depend only on the song to give position.

2. When this seems secure, ask the patient to name and touch parts of the body before singing the song.

3. Gradually depend less and less on the song, until eventually the patient can perform the task successfully independently of the music.

The restless patient is a frequent problem in geriatric work, whether in a hospital unit or nursing home, and music may give some assistance. Basically, one adopts the behaviour modification techniques that have been successfully used in the United States by music therapists to change behaviour patterns in children who are hyperactive. A resume of one such case will indicate the techniques adopted, which—in a modified form—might be applied in geriatric care.

The child concerned was very restless, and the intention of the music therapy was to teach her to remain playing quietly with her toys in a given part of the house. The child was sufficiently fond of music for this to be used as reinforcement in the teaching process. As long as the child stayed in the prescribed area (drawn as a circle on the floor of the observation room in the music therapy department), music was played on a hidden loudspeaker; as soon as the child became hyperactive or destructive, the music was switched off by the unseen therapist in the next room who was watching proceedings through a one-way observation window. Gradually, the child's behaviour pattern was altered, becoming more controlled and less restless.[5] In another case involving a woman, similar results were obtained, and as the woman became more conscious of her own behaviour she found that she was able to control her own restlessness merely by thinking of music.

Clearly a nursing home would not have the sophisticated equipment used in the work described above. However, by repeatedly telling a patient that the music will be switched off if he keeps moving around in a manner which is generally disturbing, one may approximate the results obtained above. It is important, of course, that one should not use empty threats. If one says that a given behaviour will result in music being switched off, one must make sure that this does in fact happen. If new patterns of behaviour are to be learned, the conditions must be consistent. In such a change of behaviour, one may be making use of what is called insightful learning—that is, the sudden change in behaviour which takes place because of what has been learned in a similar situation in the past. There might be insightful learning in old age as the result of learning in childhood that when music was played at a concert, one had to sit quietly to show good manners.

One may readily see that learning is the most vital of all aspects of human behaviour, since on the ability to learn from past experience depends our survival in the world, both as individuals and as *homo sapiens*. In the geriatric unit, one may utilize much of the theoretical knowledge about learning and teaching, reinforcement, transfer of training, storage and recall, to help patients in their efforts to regain and maintain their independence. Of the methods used, music is of only minor importance in the physical context—although it may provide valuable additional stimuli and reinforcement—but appears to be of prime importance from an emotional point of view, in providing a suitable atmosphere in which optimum learning may take place.

REFERENCES

1. Champion, R. A., *Learning and Activation*, Wiley and Sons, Sydney, 1967, p. 10.
2. Edson, Lee, 'Science probes a last frontier: the brain', *Think*, I.B.M., Dec. 1970, pp. 2-8.
3. NcNulty, J. and Caird, W. 'Memory loss with age—storage or retrieval?', *Psychological Reports*, 1966, pp. 229-230.
4. Harwood, E. 'Cross-sectional appraisal of the longitudinal study known as "Operation Retirement"', *Proceedings of Sixth Annual Conference, Aust. Assn. of Gerontology*, 1970, pp. 85-8.
5. Steel, A. E. 'Programmed use of music to alter unco-operative problem behaviour', *Journal of Music Therapy*, Dec. 1968, pp. 103-7.

D

7. Music in specific conditions

MUSIC THERAPY FOR BRAIN DAMAGE AND
NEUROLOGICAL DISEASE

After the nervous system has been damaged (assuming it is the result of a single trauma or cerebrovascular accident and not of an expanding neoplasm or degenerative condition with progressive effects) the question in the minds of all concerned with rehabilitation is: *How much improvement can we expect?*

Rehabilitation has been described as 'the planned withdrawal of support'.[1] Using this definition, we can see that the possibility of withdrawing support and leaving the patient to live in an independent manner depends on the extent of amelioration which occurs in the central nervous system.

It is impossible to forecast with any great accuracy the extent of the improvement which will take place, but scales of values have been devised, especially for stroke patients, which will give an indication of the probable outcome of rehabilitation.[2] These take into account such factors as incontinence, ability to dress and feed oneself, walking and speech. So far, no scale attempts to score a patient's motivation, but the examining physician commonly makes an informal rating of this when assessing a patient for treatment in a restorative unit. Tobis gives a list of 12 questions which the physician should ask himself in evaluating the emotional and psychological state of the patient as it affects prognosis for rehabilitation.[3] These are concerned with:

the degree of confusion of the patient, attention, comprehension of instructions, concentration, memory, perceptual defects, ability to recognise his own errors, distractibility, co-operation, initiative, emotional stability, and realistic goals and outlook.

In the recovery from brain damage, Grinker and Sahs[4] list the following stages:

1. The passing off of neural shock.

2. Restitution—the lessening of oedema, hyperaemia and stasis around the lesion (in this stage, flaccid paralysis changes to spastic paralysis).

3. Recovery, in the adoption of new function and also the utilization of systems previously used as accessory media only.

These writers point out, for example, that under normal circumstances the extra-pyramidal tract acts in an accessory capacity only in control of movements, but that when the cortex is damaged, it may become entirely responsible for control apart from any adaptation of other tissues which takes place. Thus we see gross movements, such as shoulder motions, being carried out effectively, but finer movements, such as the finger actions required for playing the piano, are not possible. They also point out that the effects of brain damage are not entirely confined to the side of the body opposite to the side of the brain on which damage occurred, because some nerve fibres from the precentral gyrus do descend on the same side of the body.

Luria, the noted Russian neurologist and psychologist, has written at length on the adaptation of new cortical systems to take over control of movement[5] (apart from those which result from the use of symmetrical areas in the other hemisphere, through the crossing over of fibres via the corpus callosum) and some mention will be made of his writings in later sections of this book. Although Luria's work and that of his colleagues was done mainly with penetrating head wounds from war injuries, his findings have bearing on work with cerebrovascular accidents and other brain damage which are seen in the geriatric unit.

Long-term recovery also depends on the patient's own capacity for adapting his life to coping with disability, and the prevention of secondary disabilities such as contractures.

In the early stages of brain damage, in which the patient is described as being in the acute phase, he remains confused for some time after unconsciousness has passed. Music can be of assistance in re-orientating the patient, helping to calm his fears and confusion. A parallel may be drawn here with patients who are recovering from electroconvulsive therapy (E.C.T.), when it is found that music helps to reduce the period of confusion and disorientation. (Because of the heightened sensitivity to noise, it is important that music should be played very softly at this stage.) Although the parallel is not an exact one, there is enough in common between the post-E.C.T. states and the confused state which follows brain damage for music to be advised as therapy for both.

Because restlessness and anxiety are not conducive to healing, music may also be regarded as having a part to play in the ordinary healing processes which take place after any lesion, in lessening tensions.

We may summarize the main uses of music in the treatment of brain damage as follows:

1. Music is used to give psychological stimulation, in the setting up of a group therapy situation, and in improving motivation. It also acts as a powerful socializing agent and may provide a satisfying hobby.

2. It can aid physical therapy, giving rhythmic help in walking and other patterned activities, and with breathing.

3. It also assists in the recovery of function of paralysed limbs, in rebuilding of co-ordination, postural sense, the sense of personal and extra-personal space, and in general proprioception.

4. In problems of articulation and general speech difficulties music can help.

5. For those who are beyond rehabilitation, music provides a meaningful activity which helps to retain alertness and general activity.

Some of the problems mentioned above may seem to be solely the province of the speech therapist, but it has been found that pathology of speech is not necessarily correlated with disorientation in personal space. There are, of course, diffuse lesions in which there is a speech defect as well as the disorientation, but in some types of brain damage—as for example in Gerstmann's syndrome—there is spatial agnosia without speech pathology.[6,7] In such cases the problem may escape detection, but the routine use of action songs which involve the use of 'left and right' will show up any such problem. In lesions which do involve speech defects, the ideal situation is to have a combined program of therapy, such as is used in the Geriatric Hospital at Hilversum, Holland, in which all initial treatment of aphasia is approached through the use of music, and music and speech therapy are seen as complementary activities. Such co-operation is especially necessary in any exercise which involves the naming of the digits: a patient who has learned to play the piano will always think of the thumb as being his first finger, because it is so numbered in piano music (except for a few old continental publications), but to the speech therapist, the index finger is regarded as the first finger—and rightly so, on physiological grounds. The confusion to the patient if a uniform approach is not adopted can be imagined.

It is a well-known phenomenon that many aphasiacs can sing, and in a recent article in *Gerontologia Clinica* (Vol. 13, No. 5, 1971), Hurwitz suggests that this should not be regarded as merely a neurological oddity, but that musical phrases might be endowed with meaning and used as a means of communication for the aphasiac. His paper ends with the words 'To sing and to communicate is a consummation to be desired in the aphasiac.'

In any country such as Australia, which has an extensive migration program, foreign patients will be met who have become aphasic as the result of brain damage. As Lord Brain pointed out in his authoritative work on the diseases of the nervous system, it is not always the acquired language which is obliterated; the mother tongue may be lost and the acquired language retained.[8] One may use music to test this, the reaction to songs of the homeland and to songs of the new country may give some indication of which language remains. Lord Brain also advocated the use of musical stimuli in order to raise the physiological level of the speech centres in the brain.

Parkinson's disease is often encountered in a geriatric unit. The most clearly seen features of the disease are the forward-leaning posture, the slow and difficult movements, the expressionless face, and—in many cases—tremor. In the past, references have been made to a separate category of arteriosclerotic parkinsonism, characterised by rigidity rather than tremor.[9] In 1964, however, Eadie and Sutherland published a survey of the literature and an account of an investigation into this matter, matching a group of 96 Parkinson patients with a control group of 96 orthopaedic patients.[10] The incidence of arterial disease was found to be the same in both groups, showing the unlikelihood of arteriosclerosis being a prime cause of Parkinsonism. In 1968, Selby also wrote of the low correlation between arterial disease and Parkinson's disease, and referred to the 'fundamental enigma' of the condition.[11] It is necessary to recognise that despite its name *paralysis agitans* or 'shaking palsy', Parkinson's disease is not always characterised by tremor, and it is important to take the presenting features of each patient into account when planning activities— 'Parkinson' patients are rarely able to play the piano.

Because the symptoms of the disease are commonly aggravated by emotional disturbance and tension, music can help the patient by aiding relaxation.[12] In the small unit, in which only a very few cases of the disease may be treated on any one day, the use of music in therapy will be limited to relaxation and the provision of a pleasant hobby to be followed at home in the purposeful listening to music, and—in those' whose speech is not gravely affected—in the discussion of their problems in a group setting.

In a larger department, where there may be a separate group of 'Parkinsonism' patients, music may be used as accompaniment to physical activity in relaxing mental tension. Thus the treatment may prove more effective, whether it consists of passive movements to ease rigidity or the training of new methods of walking, such as learning to turn in a large circle instead of abruptly in a 'V' turn.

With the coming of L-dopa and amantadine, the life of many sufferers from Parkinson's disease has been radically altered, but even with patients who have greatly benefited from the new drug regimes, the author has found that music has a part to play in reestablishing confidence in their own ability to move, especially with those for whom mental confusion is an added hazard.

Because of the characteristic development of dementia, the inheritance-linked disease of Huntington's Chorea is usually seen only in psycho-geriatric departments, but the few who do not develop dementia may be seen in the ordinary geriatric unit.[13] Because of the distressing involuntary movements, the release movements typical of an extra-pyramidal involvement, little can be done by the music therapist for sufferers from this disease, apart from psychological support in playing the patient's favourite tunes and trying as much as possible to understand what he says and reply to his remarks. In some cases, the ability to sing a tune (but without any recognizable vowels or consonants) is retained to a remarkable degree. The author worked with one such patient who, on the day before he died, was still able to sing, approximately, his favourite songs when they were played to him, even though his movements were so violent that it took three male nurses to give him a drink. (The violence is involuntary, not malicious.) In giving such patients a sense of achievement in the singing of their favourite songs, we are truly using music as a therapeutic activity.

In the degenerative disease of multiple sclerosis (there is no present cure) the purpose of therapy is to help the patient make best use of the resources remaining to him, and to use the characteristic remissions—firstly to live life as normally as possible during these remissions, and secondly to prepare for the next stage of the disease in the building up of proprioceptive techniques. The special techniques used in the treatment of this disease are called proprioceptive neuromuscular facilitation, or P.N.F. The particular problems of the illness in which music may help are those of breathing and voice control, and percussion band instruments, carefully selected, may be used to improve both grasp and release as well as co-ordination. It is possible that proprioceptive techniques may validly be used in the treatment of multiple sclerosis, but at present this is a matter of supposition only.

Not all victims of this disease exhibit the characteristic euphoria—some become very frustrated and depressed, and for them music should be used in an attempt to elevate the mood. The relaxation which may be induced by music can also help to alleviate the spasticity of muscles.[14]

ORTHOPAEDIC DISABILITIES

As will be realised from its name, the specialty of orthopaedics was originally concerned with congenital deformities, but today the field is far wider. The deformities dealt with have their origin in a wide variety of diseases and trauma. So varied are they that little definite use of music can be suggested, except insofar as the pain of rehabilitation is concerned.

Fear of pain can be a limiting factor in treatment, especially when movement of joints is involved. Many of the aged show a very low pain threshold, and by relaxing the patient one may raise this threshold sufficiently for the necessary techniques to be used by the physiotherapist. Startling proof of this was seen with a patient who had sustained a severe cerebrovascular thrombosis and was very much afraid of the pain she thought would result from the passive moving of the involved arm by the physiotherapist. The patient's attention was distracted by the playing of a musical instrument to one side of her, and was held by discussion of the songs being played while the physiotherapist raised the paralysed arm to shoulder height. The patient showed no sign of pain, nor indeed of awareness of what was being done. When she saw where her arm was she immediately felt pain, but until that moment had not felt any such sensation. Obviously this type of work cannot be done as a routine measure, unless one has unlimited personnel, but it might be done occasionally, if only to show the patient what can be accomplished.

Although not a matter of deformity, it seems appropriate to

discuss here the problems of gait which are often seen in the aged, and which contribute greatly to their social isolation in making it hard for them to get about and may even foster the development of disuse disabilities and contractures.[15] Loss of confidence, general anxiety and fear, possible deterioration of proprioception—all of these can be responsible for the different types of faulty gait which are seen in a geriatric unit:

1. The tottering gait of tiny steps, with the top half of the body well in advance of the centre of gravity, usually accompanied by cries of alarm, the *timor decandendi* referred to by Agate.

2. The backward leaning gait.

3. The gait in which the feet appear to be held to the floor by magnetic attraction.

4. The festinating gait of the patient with Parkinsonism, in which the problem is to get going, after which the patient may actually run with tiny steps.

All these are very real barriers to the normal, everyday way of life. By giving a feeling of relaxation and, in a sense, distracting the patient from what he is doing, as well as establishing a rhythmic response, music can accomplish much in the treatment of problems of gait in the elderly. (It has been successfully used in this way in the treatment of children in Ireton Hall School, which deals mainly with children suffering from cerebral palsy.)[16]

RESPIRATORY DISEASES

The idea of employing music in the treatment of respiratory conditions has a long history. William Byrd (1542-1623), in the preface to his *Psalmes Sonnets and Songs of Sadness and Piete*, wrote:

The exercise of singing is delightful to Nature and good to preserve the health of Man.

It doth strengthen all parts of the brest, and doth open the pipes. It is a singular good remedie for stutting and stammering in the speech.

In a later century, Quantz, the flute teacher and performer whose works and teachings are still regarded as authoritative today, wrote that 'playing the flute is "salutary and beneficial; it expands and strengthens the chest" '.[17]

In the treatment of asthma, the study of a wind instrument is commonly prescribed by physicians. The benefit is twofold: first the psychological one derived from achievement (and in a disease which has strong possibilities of being psychogenic in origin, the psychological boost to the morale is of particular value), and secondly the physical factor of learning breath control in an un-emotional setting, in which the techniques of breathing are learned primarily in order to make music and not just to mitigate an attack of asthma. It is important, of course, that the musical instrument should be suitable. The oboe, for example, in which one of the difficulties of performance lies in the small amount of air used in playing, and in getting rid of the excess air at the end of a musical phrase, would probably not be a suitable study, nor would the obtaining of an *embouchure* (proper mouth shape and position) in the French horn be easy for a very tense individual. But the flute or its near relative the recorder are most appropriate, given an understanding teacher who is interested in problems of the personality as well as in producing good performers. The recorder is commonly used overseas in schools such as the Wilson Stuart School near Birmingham, U.K., for treatment of asthma or of children with other respiratory handicaps. The clarinet too, in which even quite young children can often produce a satisfying tone, managing the correct *embouchure* without difficulty, would be suitable for even a tense person.

For chair-bound patients, or any whose disability is marked, musical accompaniments to the necessary breathing exercises add to the enjoyment and performance of the exercises, establishing rhythm and persistence. (But care must be taken not to allow patients to be over-oxygenated in their enthusiasm!) (see page 85.)

A certain case of emphysema seen in a ward of a general hospital gives a good example of motivation in respiratory conditions. The patient was lying on his side, with an oxygen mask over his face, and the sister remarked in an undertone that his prognosis was almost nil. However, on hearing the sound of music, the patient removed the oxygen mask, half sat up, and remarked that he wouldn't waste time breathing in oxygen if he could be singing instead—and this he did, with significant benefit both physically and psychologically.

THE TREATMENT OF THE CONFUSED, THE SENILE AND THE PSYCHOTIC

In his book on *The Practice of Geriatrics*, Agate comments on the need for careful distinction between the different degrees of mental deterioration, and for more careful use of the terms describing the conditions listed above.[15] However, in their reactions to music, confused, senile and psychotic patients have much in common. For reasons already mentioned, music gets through to people who are otherwise inaccessible. Temporarily it will calm and re-orientate the confused and the senile; it will distract psychotic patients from destructive and aggressive behaviour, or from their hallucinations and obsessions. (Such reactions are not entirely predictable, but are seen in many patients.) Music should be routine in the treatment and care of mental disorder.

MUSIC FOR THE BLIND

Those who have become blind late in life present special problems: they seldom gain the confidence and mobility achieved by those who are blind from birth or who lose their sight at a relatively early age when they are still able to adapt themselves appropriately to their environment. The elderly tend to be fearful of moving around, the bogy of a fractured femur haunting their steps. When financial or family circumstances have forced them to move away from their familiar surroundings, then their timidity is the worse. In the education of blind children, music is extensively used to assist confidence and rhythm in moving, and for the aged, musical accompaniment may be used similarly to allay anxiety and to promote a steady and purposeful gait. It is, however, often impossible to overcome the natural fears of the elderly blind, and their lack of confidence accentuates the social isolation and boredom so often the lot of even the sighted elderly person.

Some ageing people can learn Braille, and make use of the various activities based on tactile sensation which are designed for the blind—e.g. playing cards and dominoes with raised 'pips'. But in old age, the ability to learn a new skill is often diminished, either because of emotional reactions to disability or because of intellectual impairment. Furthermore, a significant number of those who have become blind late in life have lost their sight through *diabetes mellitus,* and of these many have—as the result of this disease—lost the acute sensitivity of the fingertips necessary for the successful use of braille notation and kindred activities.

For all the blind, but particularly for those mentioned above, it is essential to build up a satisfying way of life, to compensate in some measure for the loss of sight and to give a source of aesthetic, intellectual and social stimulation—music may help.

All broadcasting stations play recordings of different types, varying from 'pop' music, through the semi-serious musicals to the most serious of classical and contemporary compositions. It is possible to obtain details of what music is to be played by most stations, either in printed program guides issued in magazine-type publications, or in the columns of the newspapers. When a sighted person is available to read and discuss these programs, then listening can be planned ahead in a purposeful way and a genuine hobby created. It may also be possible to obtain 'talking books' from the local organization for the blind, to enable the blind to hear biographies of composers or books about music.

But even if the blind person is thrown entirely on his own resources in planning his listening to music, he will find that he becomes familiar with the times and content (in general terms) of regular broadcasts, knowing that at one time of day, opera is performed, at another light piano music, and so on. Since regular comperes are often assigned to regular series of broadcasts, the listener will often build up a sense of familiarity with the voice and personality of the compere of each series, and when there are broadcasters of the calibre of the late Walford Davies a surprising warmth of feeling is created for the personality of the speaker. This is, of course, but a poor substitute for real person-to-person relationships, but it is better than nothing in alleviating loneliness and monotony.

Discussing music can also provide a common interest between the blind and the sighted, and one in which the blind may even excel. This is not because, as is sometimes asserted, the hearing of the blind is necessarily the more acute, but because the blind, in depending so much on audible stimuli to interpret the world around them, have to make the best possible use of their auditory potential and thus may seem to be more acute of hearing than those for whom auditory and visual cues have more or less equal importance.

For the performer of music who loses his sight, there will be satisfaction in playing again the works enjoyed in the past, and for some it may be possible to learn Braille musical notation in order to study new and unfamiliar works. (The telephone directory will provide information regarding the whereabouts of the local organization for the blind, through which it should be possible to arrange for the provision of tuition in braille etc., as well as, in most places, for talking books to be brought or sent.)

Operating a record player is a relatively easy skill to acquire, and one which will open the way to much enjoyment of music. It will be necessary to devise some means of classifying and marking the records so that the blind person can choose what to play.

By writing on the record sleeve with a hard ballpoint (removing the record first for safety), it is possible to make a good label which can be interpreted fairly readily by the blind, or, if an embossed tape machine is available, a sighted friend or relative could label all the records. In some areas, lending libraries have a section for recorded music, and it should be possible to borrow these for the blind.

For the partially sighted, books are available in large print, and the Ulverscroft range of large-print books includes books about music and musicians as well as hymn books and other song books.

Although nothing can entirely compensate for the aged's loss of sight, music may help to alleviate the unhappiness which such a loss brings, and even those who, in earlier life, had no time or inclination for listening to serious music, may develop such an interest under their changed circumstances, given encouragement and help from therapists and family.

LONG-STAY AND TERMINAL CARE

In every nursing home there will be found a large number of patients for whom rehabilitation has long since ceased to be feasible, and for whom only long-term nursing care can be provided. In most hospitals today, patients' records will be found to include the direction 'T.L.C.', which stands for Tender Loving Care, and this indicates the comparatively modern realization that physical care is not enough. For the total care of a patient he must be made aware that people care *about* him as well as caring *for* him in a nursing sense. In many nursing homes, such T.L.C. is given without any need for a doctor to order it, but nevertheless there are many instances in which an extra 'dose' can be a great benefit in helping the patient over some extra stress, as in bereavement of friends and relatives or a further stroke. Sometimes one sees neglect of aged relatives by their families, who stop coming to visit the patient, and in this crisis again extra doses of Tender Loving Care must be given. Not that this can atone for neglect, but it will help the patient to keep his self-respect despite the lack of interest from those who should care about his happiness.

A recent study on the use of the drug cinnarizine, described in *Gerentologia Clinica*,[18] gives an interesting demonstration of the response of even the apparently hopeless patient to an interest in his or her welfare. The patients concerned in the double-blind study consisted of fifty women, with an average age of eighty-three, living in four different hospitals. All of them suffered from the effects of multiple cerebrovascular accidents, all were frail and all except three showed marked mental deterioration. In seventeen, the degree of dementia was regarded as gross. It had therefore been expected that there would be results, positively or negatively, only from the drug itself and that no placebo effect would be seen. However, it was found that there was a marked placebo effect, and that in all groups, in all hospitals, the patients did better with the placebo than with the drug being tested. The experiment was designed only to test the efficacy or otherwise of cinnarizine, but did, unintentionally, also demonstrate that no patient should be regarded as being too far gone in age or disability to respond to an active interest in his or her well-being.

The provision of musical activities in long-stay and terminal wards is one way of showing such an interest. On entering a long-stay ward with a musical instrument, such as a piano-accordion or a portable organ, one notices an immediate stir—the rustling of bedclothes, the moving of feet of those who are up, other indescribable signs of increased activity. This is partly the result of someone coming into the room, but is mainly due to the music itself. A record player produces some increase in activity, but less than is seen when an instrument is actually played.

One of the major problems in the nursing of the bedridden is the avoidance of pressure sores, and Exton-Smith[19] and others have, by fixing measuring devices to the beds of long-stay patients, assessed a correlation between the number of spontaneous movements made and the incidence of pressure sores. While it would be foolish to suggest that having music played in a terminal-care ward would remove all danger of pressure sores, there is a grain of truth in the idea. This is so because the stimulating effects of the music do not cut off when the music ceases. It has been observed in long-stay wards and in semi-invalid groups that the general level of activity is increased for some time after the music session has finished. Indeed, in one psychogeriatric ward it has been noted by the charge nurse that a weekly sing-song and band session has encouraged the singing of songs on other days, and has also helped to keep the patients orientated in time, in remembering which day to expect 'The Music Lady'. The same charge nurse has reported that nurses coming from other wards where music is not, so far, a regular feature of the program notice a difference in atmosphere and attribute it to the spontaneous singing which often occurs. One medical officer was surprised when a patient who had difficulty in remembering even his own name remarked 'Music Lady will be here soon, Doctor, half-past ten she comes.' And this was from a patient for whom music was a once-a-week-only event.

For patients who are in a nursing home only on account of a physical disability, and who remain alert, it is highly necessary to provide intellectual stimulation. In some nursing homes, newspaper and other discussion groups are a regular feature, and it is worth while considering also the establishment of musical discussion programs, the records to be chosen by patients if possible. Dr Harwood[20] of Queensland University has written of the value for the elderly of undertaking a definite course of study. Some of the enthusiastic members of a study program in German (as a new language) who were successful in the examination were in their eighties. The serious study of music could likewise prove a most worthwhile occupation.

Even in terminal wards where patients are suffering severe pain, music seldom causes any distress, but, on the contrary, is enjoyed as offering temporary distraction from bodily pain. Partly, this is because the music is dispensed by a visible person— music from a loudspeaker would not represent the same personal interest—but partly the effects are due to the three-fold nature of the music itself: in stimulating the mind, relaxing the body and comforting the spirit.

In long-stay care, one has not only the basic cause of the patient's illness to deal with, but also the results of inactivitiy. Disuse syndromes have already been dealt with in part—e.g. pressure sores—but there are a few others which should be mentioned here. Hirschberg, Lewis and Thomas' book on rehabilitation gives clear lists of such syndromes,[21] listing them by cause, condition produced and prevention. Of these, several might be either prevented or mitigated by music therapy—for instance, muscle atrophy caused by insufficient exercise. Simple exercises, performed in bed or chair with a strong rhythmical accompaniment, would help to prevent disuse syndromes.

Certain circulatory disturbances, under which hypostatic pneumonia may be included, could likewise be assisted by a program of musically-based exercises. As anecdotal evidence of patients' attitude, the following incident is relevant: An elderly man said that he thought the music program was 'great'—'You feel like giving up. Then you hear the music and say to yourself, O well, I'll give it another go!'

Exercise programs should include work with sphincter muscles, the music assisting the 'holding in' time for this work (see page 81). It is interesting to note that, in the lists of disuse syndromes mentioned above, psychological deterioration is included, as being caused by separation (and therefore disuse) from normal social interaction and by increasing depersonalization through hospital routine. The writers referred to advocate the active participation of patients in planning the activities as being a means of preventing such deterioration.

REFERENCES

1. Hyams. D. E. 'Psychological factors in rehabilitation of the elderly', *Gerontologia Clinica*, vol. 11, no. 3, 1969, pp. 129-139.
2. Wylie, C. M. 'Gauging the response of stroke patients to rehabilitation, *Journal of The American Geriatrics Society*, vol. XV, no. 9, 1967.
3. Tobis, E. *Evaluation and Management of The Brain-Damaged Patient*, Thomas, Springfield, 1960, p. 42.
4. Grinker, R. and Sahs, A. *Neurology* (6th edn.), Thomas, Springfield, 1966, pp. 128 and 612.
5. Luria, A. *The Restoration of Function After Brain Injury*, Pergamon, Oxford, 1963, p. 45. (Originally published in Russian by Medgiz, Moscow, titled *Vosstanovlenie funktsi mozga posle voyennoi travmy*.)
6. Semmes, J. *et al.* 'Correlates of impaired orientation in personal and extrapersonal space', *Brain*, vol. 86, pt. 4, Dec. 1963, pp. 474-82.
7. Gerstmann. J. 'Some notes on Gerstmann's syndrome', *Neurology*, no. 7, Dec. 1957, pp. 866-9.
8. Brain, Lord *Diseases of the Nervous System*, (6th edn.), Oxford University Press, 1962, p. 186.
9. *Ibid.* p. 478.
10. Eadie, M. J. and Sutherland, J. M. 'Arteriosclerosis in Parkinson's disease', *Journal of Neurology, Neurosurgery and Psychiatry*, vol. 27, 1964, pp. 237-240.
11. Selby G. 'Parkinson's disease', in *Handbook of Clinical Neurology*, (eds.) Vincken and Bruyn, North Holland, Amsterdam, 1968, pp. 183-207.
12. Brain, *op. cit.*, p. 475.
13. Walsh, F. *Diseases of the Nervous System*, Livingstone, London, 1963, p. 29.
14. Brain, *op. cit.*, p. 457.
15. Agate, J. *The Practice of Geriatrics*, (2nd edn.) Heinemann, London, p. 285, p. 357.
16. Lubran, A. *Music Therapy and The Spastic Child*, British Society for Music Therapy, 1960.
17. Quantz, J. J. *On Playing The Flute*, Faber and Faber, London, 1966, p. 27 (originally published 1752).
18. Irvine, R. E. *et al.* 'Cinnarizine in cerebrovascular disease', *Gerontologia Clinica*, vol. 12, no. 5, 1970, pp. 297-301.
19. Exton-Smith, A. N. and Sherwood, R. W. 'Prevention of pressure sores', *Lancet*, Nov. 1961, p. 1124-26.
20. Harwood, E. 'Cross-sectional appraisal of the longitudinal study known as "Operation Retirement"', *Proceedings of Sixth Annual Conference, Aust. Assn. of Gerontology*, 1970, pp. 85-8.
21. Hirschberg, G., Lewis, L. and Thomas. D. *Rehabilitation*, Lippincott, Philadelphia, 1964, p. 15.

8. Contraindications

It must never be assumed that music has universal applications in therapy, either in psychiatric work or in geriatric work. Fortunately, the number of people for whom music is either undesirable or definitely contraindicated is few, but such cases must not be ignored merely because of their small numbers.

MUSICOGENIC EPILEPSY

There is a comparatively rare but well-documented condition known as *musicogenic epilepsy*, in which music, generally of a certain frequency, 'triggers' the particular brain pattern which causes an epileptic seizure.[1] For patients suffering from this condition, exclusion from music sessions is essential. It is realized that in the course of daily life the chances are that they will occasionally hear music unintentionally—especially since these days people play background music on every conceivable occasion and in every imaginable place—but there is no point in exposing them unnecessarily to the possibility of further attacks. It should, however, be recognized that there are many patients who have epileptic attacks during a music session, attacks not caused by the music; they are people who have many attacks each day, and would in all probability have had the seizure under consideration whether attending a music group or not. Since boredom appears to be a precipitating cause of attacks in idiopathic epilepsy, any activity which reduces the monotony of existence should be promoted, not forbidden.[2]

BOREDOM, DISLIKE OF MUSIC

Although tone-deafness as an actual defect of hearing, in which the person cannot distinguish high or low tones, is a rarity, those who find it hard to distinguish a melody will not enjoy listening to music. Most of those people who say that they are tone-deaf, and have in childhood been excluded from school or church choirs, are in fact unable to co-ordinate what they hear with the sound which they produce with their vocal apparatus. The ear has usually not been cultivated to listen with accuracy, and so we get the phenomenon usually described as 'the growler', the individual who cannot sing in tune with anyone else and who is often only marginally aware of his unpitched singing. (The truly tone-deaf is distinguished by a monotonous speaking voice, which strikes the listener as being a dull, dead tone.) The growler has usually been ignored by the school teacher, even though the condition can be remedied in most cases by education in listening and muscular co-ordination. Frequently the growler has also been humiliated by these failures, made to feel an unco-operative fool. It has been estimated that some 6 per cent of the British population is tone deaf,[3] with a physical tissue defect to account for the condition. People who have difficulty in perceiving differences in pitch are not likely to have enjoyed music at school, and so, even in an adult, hospital setting, music may still have unhappy associations for them. Such people should not be expected to join in music sessions if their first attendance proves truly distasteful to them, although one may be able to uncover reasons for dislike of music and change the attitude once the patient has recognised the reasons for his dislike.

EMOTIONAL DISTURBANCE

The problem of the tearful patient has already been discussed earlier in some detail. In general, it is not desirable to exclude the tearful patient whose grief is quietly expressed. There may, however, be emotionally upset patients whose grief, tears, etc., are noisy and who disturb the rest of the group. The best course is probably to allow the rest of the group to decide whether they wish the patient concerned to remain or temporarily to be excluded until the reasons for the behaviour have been sorted out. Some groups of people can be very supportive to an unhappy member; others have so many antagonistic feelings that the presence of the weeping patient seriously jeopardises the success of the activity. The exclusion should, nevertheless, be regarded as a temporary measure, unless the tears and disturbance are from an organic brain syndrome or other condition which does not admit of significant improvement. And even with the organic brain syndrome, it is possible, as Inskip suggested,[4] that we over-generalise about the difficulties of dealing with this condition, that a

B

vital consideration in the constructive treatment and rehabilitation of such patients is the frustration tolerance of the therapist and the degree of self-knowledge and maturity which he/she attains, as well as the more usually considered variables of the *patient's* condition.

OTHER CONSIDERATIONS

Patients who have feelings of persecution, whether part of a psychosis or not, should be handled carefully, and if possible given only praise in the early stages of their participation in musical work (and indeed in any work). Later, if it is necessary to suggest ways in which they might improve the quality of their work, care should be taken that any comments are made in private and with as much opportunity for face-saving as possible.

Depressed patients, for whom the condition has assumed the proportions of a psychosis, usually have very marked guilt feelings about their condition. We may be able to help them by giving them the chance to serve the community in some measure—for example, in tidying the room after a music session, putting books and instruments away. For those with marked mood-swings, the inevitability of such swings must be accepted. We must never allow ourselves to succumb to the temptation of thinking, 'Mrs X is being difficult today. She could easily do whatever is required if she wanted to.' Most of us have the experience of feeling slightly 'blue' for no definable reason, and there are many degrees of this, from the normal—which we all assume ourselves to be—to the abnormal manic-depressive psychosis, with almost innumerable states in between. For patients who exhibit these tendencies, we must be alert for signs that the mood has changed, and adapt our techniques of handling them accordingly. For example, in the manic phase, many patients show marked aggression which is exacerbated by the use of such aggressive-type musical instruments as cymbals. Far from calming them by externalising their hostility, the use of such instruments tends to provoke still more aggressive, destructive behaviour. In the depressive phase, on the other hand, one sees a fear of noisy instruments, and the same guilty feeling mentioned above. Here we must again give the patient the opportunity to work out his feelings by serving the group, which gives him the feeling of expiating his guilt. (Despite, of course, there being in fact no guilt to expiate.)

It may be thought that such elaborate details regarding dealing with psychoses are unnecessary in a book devoted to what might be called normal geriatric care—that patients who required such careful handling, with so much consideration for psychiatric factors, would be in an institution for the mentally ill and not in nursing homes and geriatric wards. However, the survey of the Newcastle-on-Tyne area in Britain, already referred to, shows that in the area concerned this was not so. (And there is no logical reason for the situation being different anywhere else, there being no special reason why Newcastle-on-Tyne should have a high number of cases of mental illness.) The statistics from this survey showed that a significant proportion of the elderly with mental diseases are being cared for either at home, or in nursing homes and geriatric wards. It is therefore appropriate that some comments should be given on the handling, in a musical milieu, of those who have quite marked mental disturbance.

OVER-SENSITIVITY TO NOISE AS A CONTRAINDICATION

After brain damage of any kind, there is sometimes a sensitivity to noise, which includes even music of a normal volume. Since in a geriatric unit there will be many patients whose hearing is impaired, the volume at which music is played is often louder than average, and so these sensitive patients will be still more likely to find the playing of records, or even singing, worrisome. The solution to this problem is to seat the patients at a distance from the music, since they do not usually dislike music as such but merely the volume of sound. At times, it may even be necessary to seat the patient in the garden, outside the window, but such extreme measures will seldom be necessary for long, and one can gradually bring the patient nearer, at first placing him at the end of the room or in the doorway to the corridor, and gradually putting him nearer and nearer until he is at the edge of the group.

REFERENCES

1. Merritt, H. H. *Textbook of Neurology*, (2nd edn.), Lea and Febiger, Philadelphia, 1959, p. 683.
2. Maddison, D., Day, P. and Leabeater, B. *Psychiatric Nursing*, Livingstone, London, 1963, p. 266.
3. Cox, I. *Psychological Abstracts*, vol. 22, no. 9, Sept. 1948: Abstract 3705 on tone-deafness, describing work done by Dennis Fry, Physical Society, London.
4. Inskip, W. 'Treatment programs for patients with chronic brain syndrome can be successful', *Journal of The American Geriatrics Society*, vol. XVIII, 1970, pp. 631-6.

9. *The future—possible developments and fields of research*

In all the literature of music therapy, there are more anecdotes about its value than evidence gained from planned experimental work.

If music therapy is to be regarded as being of genuine medical value, it is important that we should be as scientific as possible in our approach to our work, lest it be thought that we fall into the *post hoc ergo propter hoc* brand of sophistry.

There are very real difficulties in following a scientific method, chief among which are those of:

1. Cross-matching individuals in order to have a control group against which to check the validity of experimental work.

2. Measuring work done.

Even with such a simple condition as a broken leg, it would be hard to find simultaneously available two subjects/patients with identical fractures, identical age, identical conditions under which the fracture was sustained, identical medical history (as influencing prognosis as to rates of healing, etc.). How much harder, then, to match up identical subjects when one is dealing with conditions such as arteriosclerosis, cerebrovascular accidents, Parkinson's disease and other conditions commonly encountered in geriatric units.

Are we then forced to follow unscientific methods, to accept as inevitable doubts which may be cast on the validity of our conclusions by workers in fields more readily open to objective measurement? Not entirely so. The difficulties we meet are not exclusive to music therapists. Similar ambiguities and weaknesses are found in much experimental work in human psychology and psychiatry, when—because of temperamental differences between individuals—one often suspects that so-called control groups are far from being genuinely equivalent to the experimental group.

Although it is undoubtedly hard to reproduce conditions exactly and then alter only one variable, what we can do in accounts of our work is to make it clear that we are aware of the *desirability* of correct cross-matching and of changing only one variable at a time, and also that we do not believe that one case adequately tests an hypothesis.

Two examples may help to clarify this point:

1. In a male public ward of a general hospital, one patient was receiving music therapy for a severe respiratory condition. The sister in charge commented spontaneously that the music was affecting everyone in the ward, making the men more cheerful and alert. In order to test whether it was in fact the music having this effect or whether it was due to the presence of a new person in the ward, the therapist went into the ward at the customary time of day, but without the piano-accordion. No particular interest was shown by the patients, and no change in posture or alteration in general level of activity occurred. As far as could be ascertained, conditions on the no-music day were identical with conditions on the previous day, namely,

    (a) Nursing shifts were the same, so the same nurses were on duty,

    (b) The time of day was the same, so—as the same amount of time had elapsed since lunch—there was no reason for patients to be sleepier.

    (c) Except for one discharge, the patient population was the same.

    (d) Nobody's condition was markedly different on the no-music day (i.e. there was nobody whose condition might have depressed the ward morale).

    (e) The weather (which can affect reactions) was the same as the day before.

From all these considerations, it seemed justifiable to conclude that the ward sister was correct—that it was the music itself which had affected the atmosphere.

2. One morning a group of psychogeriatric patients, usually very responsive to music, proved almost entirely unresponsive. Since the ward population had not changed from the week before, one might have been justified in concluding that the patients had become bored with music and needed a change of activity. However, a nurse's comment that patients had been given medication later than usual the night before and that no one had woken up properly yet made it clear that the condition

which had changed was not the patients' interest in music but the fortuitous circumstance of late bedtime sedation.

In both these examples, the alteration of one factor markedly altered the patients' response to the therapist's presence. Thus it will be seen that in all accounts of our work, we must state how many variables were the same in each episode we describe, and what steps we took either to obtain a control group or at least to obtain uniform conditions.

In all pioneer work, we must be sure that we are not suffering from what has been called the 'rose-coloured spectacles syndrome' —i.e. that because we want and expect our work to succeed, we tend to notice those things which support our hypothesis and not see those things which tend to disprove it. In other words, we must be seen as being sufficiently secure in our discipline to attain academic integrity and not to be swayed by wishful thinking.

How many cases can be said to establish and prove an hypothesis? How can we be sure that the experiment we design is in fact testing what we set out to test, and not some other undetected factor? These and many other questions can be answered only by a study of statistics, and in particular a study of those areas of statistics which deal with random sampling, the testing of experimental data and so on. It is customary today for the experimenter to work with a statistician, so that experimental conditions may be correctly planned from the outset, but in order to work intelligently with such a specialist, it is desirable for the music (or other) therapist to have some outline of knowledge of the subject, in order to appreciate what is implied in the terms used—e.g. probability curve, standard deviation, mean and median. Any good encyclopaedia will give a fair coverage of these topics, but if more detail is desired there is a wide variety of texts available, of varying degrees of difficulty.[1]

It is appropriate to quote here the eminent physiologist, L. J. Henderson on the three ingredients essential for building a science:[2] intimate contact and an habitual intuitive familiarity with the phenomena; means for systematically collecting and ordering data; an effective way of thinking about the phenomena. Consideration of such principles is equally important whether we are considering music therapy as a science or the intricacies of nuclear physics.

In what directions may we develop music therapy, either in a practical way or in planned research? The answer lies partly in our individual interests and enthusiasms.

1. For nursing staff who are worried about the apathy and withdrawal which can be such a marked feature of nursing home life, the interest will probably lie in music as a socializing factor.

2. Social workers and psychiatrists may see music's chief function as a stimulus to the talking over of problems, and a help in socialising the solitary.

3. The physiotherapist may visualise the possibilities of using music to improve performance, understanding and persistence in certain rhythmic exercises, and the rebuilding of proprioception.

4. The occupational therapist will probably see music chiefly as a means to recreation, as a diversional therapy and group activity, and also as a form of psychological stimulation.

5. The speech therapist will use music as an aid to articulation and phonation, and as a psychological boost to the morale for the aphasic patient.

6. The clinical psychologist will be able to use music as a 'trigger' to the memory, and in re-establishing impaired perception, as well as in musically-oriented discussion work.

7. The geriatrician will be able to see music as entering into all the facets of his work, and of those specialties which come under his aegis, as well as helping in the maintaining of the patient's status as an individual.

In all these suggestions it is not intended, of course, that every one of the specialist workers mentioned will necessarily want to use music. Our personal interests and gifts are clearly a decisive factor in determining how we do our work, but the list is, it is hoped, a guide to what can be done by those who *naturally* feel an interest in the therapeutic uses of music.

If music. is to enter into so many activities other than the purely musical, what can be regarded as the work which should be done by the music therapist alone? For technical reasons of training, there are some activities which the musician alone will undertake, although it must be acknowledged that there may be workers in other fields who are fully competent to undertake these (biographies of many mathematicians and scientists reveal a high degree of achievement in musical performance and knowledge). However, it is likely that music as a hobby will be 'taught' by the music therapist, who will plan record sessions and discussions, and, in any hospital where there is sufficient talent, form a choir or band. In general, these activities will be found in **psychiatric** institutions rather than geriatric units as such, but there may be large geriatric hospitals where such a range of activity is possible.

In keep-fit work and general purpose exercises, it will probably be found that the physiotherapist and the occupational therapist will be willing to leave some of the activities to the music therapist, once the basic principles and techniques have been discussed and decided upon. The music therapist will also be able to make tape-recordings of piano accompaniment for planned programs of exercises, which can be used by other personnel at times when the music therapist is not available, or when it is more convenient to use only a few minutes of accompaniment in the course of a treatment session. For remedial gymnastics performed to music, the music therapist will advise on choice of music to suit the exercises, and possibly compose appropriate music for some of these. She may also give instruction to those patients who wish to regain a lost proficiency in instrumental work, choosing pieces which will be within the patients' range of movement. At Kingsbridge Veterans' Hospital in New York, patients are frequently referred to the music therapy department for remedial work in regaining hand function as well as for improvement in breathing techniques through singing,[3] and this is common in long-stay hospitals in the U.S.A.

This brings up the question of co-operation between the various disciplines, and how this may be achieved. There are signs that the training of the various para-medical disciplines is becoming a joint venture, not only for economical reasons, but because it is being recognised more and more that the work of the disciplines must necessarily overlap, and greater ease of working will be attained if much of the training is done together. This will give each therapist an understanding of the aims and techniques of the other, and will eventually benefit the patient, since techniques will key into each other instead of, as occasionally happens, conflicting.

Another way of achieving understanding is in the setting up of study groups for the staff of rehabilitation units, in which each member of staff in turn talks about his or her own work and there is free discussion of methods adopted in this work. In one such unit, the matrons of district nursing homes also attend these sessions. It has been recommended that all staff of rehabilitation units should work through some group experiences, under guidance of a clinical psychologist, achieving by this group psychotherapy a better understanding of their own personalities, of the difficulties of working with others, of the fears and conflicts aroused by patients[4] and by other staff, and of other problems of teamwork. Ideally, all members of a therapeutic team should be sufficiently secure in their own personalities and disciplines that they can exchange roles without feeling threatened.[5] Such a state of affairs does not arise easily, and the group psychotherapy mentioned above should help to develop mature outlook and inter-personal relationships.

That the team approach to rehabilitation does work is shown by accounts such as that given in the *Journal of The American Geriatrics Society* for December 1969, in which work with a group of elderly veterans in a hospital is described. The team approach proved very successful, improving such traits as memory, attention span, perception, interest in environment and social contacts, and self-discipline.

However, it should be borne in mind that merely working together in a unit at the same time does not create a team, and that usually the hospital devoted to general medical care is less well accustomed to organisation in terms of a therapeutic community than is the psychiatric hospital. The firm hierarchical structure of many general hospitals will often not admit of such a community approach to medicine and there are very real difficulties in communication[6] between the different levels of the hospital staff. However, new hospitals which are being established, are, in many cases, being set up with a planned orientation towards the therapeutic community, so that gifts and knowledge of all staff may be best utilised, no matter what their relative position.[7] There is, of course, the problem of ultimate responsibility for the patient's progress, and in any team method of working this is a matter which must be settled. Where the music therapist fits into the general team structure varies from one place to another. In the U.S., for example, most hospitals regard all paramedical disciplines, including music therapy, as of equal value, while in a few the music therapist attains a greater dignity than his colleagues.[8] However, whatever the relative status of the music therapist, the aim should be for co-operation in treatment of patients, the patient's progress being the sole criterion by which the effectiveness of the team is measured.

Many projects can be undertaken with a team approach and although in the first instance there is an uneconomic use of staff, the results for future applications justify this.

In speech therapy, music is employed for improvement of auditory perception[9] and to establish communication,[10] but more uses could be investigated. Work is being done with brain-damaged children (e.g. at the Institute of Logopedics, Wichita, U.S.A.); it is based on the fact that music centres of the brain usually remain intact despite impairment of speech centres. By using music, statistically significant improvements are being obtained in speech and communication. Although this work is being done with children similar techniques could presumably be applied to adults (see also page 41). Nordoff and Robbins describe how rhythmic confusion in children's drum-beating indicates deep neuropsychiatric confusion.[11] This is analogous with the present author's observation (page 92) of brain-damaged adults' inability to keep time in group musical activities—this phenomenon could be investigated as a measurable indicator of patients' improvement.

Although developmental work depends on the presentation of patients, the scope of music as a therapeutic tool is broad indeed.

REFERENCES

1. Books on statistics
    (a) Cochran, W. and Cox, G. *Experimental Designs*, Wiley, New York, 1950 (esp. last chapter).
    (b) Hayslett, H. T. and Murphy, P. *Statistics Made Simple*, W. H. Allen, London, 1967.
    (c) Dverksen, G. 'Planning and understanding research', in *Music in Therapy* (ed.) Gaston, E., Macmillan, New York, 1968, p. 409.
2. Henderson, L. J. 'Essentials in building a science', in *Sociology of Small Groups*, (ed.) Mills, T., Prentice-Hall, New York, 1967, p. 25.
3. Greenbaum, D., 'Music program at Kingsbridge Veterans' Hospital', *British Journal of Music Therapy*, Autumn 1969, pp. 3-8.
4. Hirschberg, G., Lewis, L. and Thomas, D. *Rehabilitation*, Lippincott, Philadelphia, 1964, p. 59.
5. Nurcombe, B. 'Child psychiatry and the community', in *Psychiatry and The Community* (eds.) Maddison, D. and Pilowski, I., Sydney University Press, 1969, p. 123.
6. Martin, D. V. *Adventure in Psychiatry*, Cassirer, Oxford, 1962: chapter on General Hospital.
7. Norton, A. *The New Dimensions of Medicine*, Hodder and Stoughton, London, 1969, p. 133.
8. Muskatevc, L. (Ass. Prof. of Music Therapy, Univ. of Wisconsin, U.S.A.), *personal communication*.
9. Berry, M. F. and Eisenson, J. *Speech Disorders*, Peter Owen, London, 1962, p. 200.
10. *Ibid.* p. 408.
11. Nordoff, P. and Robbins, C. *Therapy in Music for Handicapped Children*, Gollancz, London, 1971, p. 57.

PRACTICAL
CONSIDERATIONS

10. *Planning music for social situations*

In planning musical work as a socialising influence, it is important to bear in mind the sensory losses of the elderly. Deficiencies of sight and hearing may be crucial to the success of the group activity.

If it is not already known, the acuteness of hearing of each patient should be assessed in an informal way, so that the patient can be placed in the group accordingly. For example, if the group is set up in a semi-circle around the piano, place those with a marked hearing deficiency in one ear next to the piano, with the good ear as near as is necessary to the side wall of the instrument. For the profoundly deaf, it will be helpful for the patient to place the hand on the side of the piano in order to feel the vibrations and thus reinforce whatever is picked up through the ear or hearing aid. For those who back up their hearing by lip-reading, place them in such a position that they can clearly see the mouth of the leader of the group, and, if possible, those of other members of the group, too.

For patients with brain damage—whether this is the result of cerebrovascular accident or other trauma—bear in mind the possibility of acute sensitivity to noise mentioned earlier, and if the patient shows marked restlessness or anxiety which is not exhibited in other situations and which can therefore be ascribed to the effects of the music, ask whether he would like to sit at the end of the room or in the passageway nearby. Generally one finds that any initial distaste for noise disappears in the patient's wish to join in the activity, and in fact a tolerance for noise may even be built up by this means, but one cannot assume that such an increase in tolerance will occur.

In some cases of hemiplaegia, there is a definite sensory loss on one side, affecting visual and auditory fields. The loss of vision sometimes escapes detection in a routine medical check, since only a part of the visual field in the eye may be lost, and the patient may not be aware of this until it is noticed that he reads only some of the words on a page. It is a good idea to be on the look-out for this type of defect, although if the patient is receiving speech therapy this will have been noted. But even without such marked deficiencies, there will probably be some sensory loss on the affected side in most cases of hemiplaegia, and it is therefore desirable to place the patient with his affected side away from the rest of the group—for example, by placing him at one end of a semi-circle, so that his 'good' side is in better contact with what is going on. When demonstrating any activity, or singing with an individual patient, one must always remember to stand on the side next to the 'good' side. (It is recognised that to use the term 'good' and 'bad' in hemiplaegia, to refer to the unaffected and affected side, is most undesirable, and in general one uses such circumlocutions as 'The stronger arm', but patients themselves usually think in terms of good and bad, and so these descriptions are used here for the sake of brevity.)

It is harder to plan group seating to compensate for defects of vision than for those of hearing, but they are the less detrimental in their effects on group relationships. The blind or partially-sighted find it easier to maintain social contacts than do the deaf, probably because nuances of verbal communication convey more information about human relationships than is the case with visual stimuli and facial expressions.

For the partially sighted, a song book has been published in large print, by the Ulverscroft Large Print Books. It has been planned with the elderly in mind. Eventually the songs in it will be out of date even for the aged, but at present anyone born up to about 1930 will be familiar with the songs included—most of them chosen by the present author.

It is encouraging, in a singing session, for patients to be able to ask for their favourite songs and have them played so that they can join in, but clearly this is not always possible. No one person can play each and every song ever written. There are three solutions to this difficulty:

1. Ask patients to plan the programs one week ahead, so that the accompanist has a chance to find the music and practise it. This diminishes the spontaneity of the activity to some extent, but is helpful as a problem-solving exercise and gives the patients some feeling of control over their own activities.

2. Encourage each person to have a second and third choice

in case the song requested cannot be found. This can have quite a therapeutic value for the demanding patient, who expects that every wish can be granted.

3. If the patient has a good enough voice to sing a recognizable melody, ask her or him to sing the tune so that the accompanist can learn it, and put a simple chord accompaniment to the tune. This can be most encouraging to the patient, helping to build up a sense of usefulness in actively contributing to the work of the group, especially if migrants can teach their native songs.

One should never be afraid to say, 'I don't know that song.' Even the senile are able to understand that no one knows all songs, and it can even be helpful in emphasising that the therapist is 'one of us', that we all have our difficulties. One must, of course, be prepared to make the same apology each week, unless one can eventually find the song requested, since many of the elderly do ask the same question over and over again without remembering the answer.

The singing of songs can be an end in itself, or it can be used as an aid to general social interaction and conversation. Questions such as 'Can you recall when you first heard this?' or, when sheet music bearing a copyright date is used, 'Would anyone like to guess when this was published?' can lead on to interesting exchange of memories. It is often necessary to draw out the more timid members, asking questions in a gentle manner. After a while, most patients welcome the chance to reminisce about events which were important to them, and it may even be necessary to restrict some if the more timid patients are feeling overwhelmed. However, it should not be assumed that all patients wish to talk about themselves at the first few sessions.

By deliberately choosing songs of a particular era, the atmosphere can, to some extent, be manipulated as may be necessary, and made livelier. For example, Irving Berlin wrote songs over more than a generation, and one may use these to build up an interesting program of parallel musical/world history. One may start with his first great success, 'Alexander's Ragtime Band', published in 1911, and go on with other of his hits right up until 'Call me Madam', in 1950, tracing the life of our civilisation through this period as running parallel with the changing styles of music, and changing lives of the patients. (Such a program can be used to initiate therapeutic discussion work, as described in the next chapter, but in the present context is intended only as a social activity.) Other Berlin song favourites widely known by most age groups (except, perhaps, those born since 1965), are 'Blue Skies', 'Always', 'White Christmas', 'Easter Parade', 'This is the Army Mr Jones', the score of 'Annie Get Your Gun', and—in the U.S. —'God Bless America'. Because of the wide popularity of this composer, his music can be used to weld together a group of patients of quite diverse ages.

Other composers of light music whose songs can be used in the same way are: **Jerome Kern** ('All the Things You Are', 'The Way You Look Tonight', 'I've Told Every Little Star', 'The Last Time I saw Paris', 'Look for the Silver Lining', songs from 'Showboat', especially 'Old Man River' and 'Smoke Gets in Your Eyes'); **Richard Rodgers** (music from 'On Your Toes,' 1936, 'Boys from Syracuse', 1938; 'Pal Joey', 1940; 'Oklahoma', 1943; 'Carousel', 1945; 'South Pacific', 1949; and 'The King and I' 1951); **George Gershwin**, whose music, although not covering such a span of years as those mentioned, is of importance in that it is appreciated by both serious and jazz musicians. His song 'Swanee', on which his early fame was founded, is still popular, and 'Rhapsody in Blue' and the music from 'Porgy and Bess' are loved by people of diverse tastes and ages. It is of interest that his musical play, 'Of Thee I Sing', was the first such play ever to win a Pulitzer Prize; **Gilbert and Sullivan**, whose operas likewise appeal to differing tastes in music and have been known and loved for many years. Simple arrangements of the favourite numbers of several of these operas are available at a reasonable cost, and are well worth buying for a geriatric unit, since they demand only a modest degree of pianistic talent to play them. They can often be played by a patient, and this is helpful to the general atmosphere of the group.

Other music around which an interesting program of listening and talking can be built are: 'The Wizard of Oz' (which may be known by two different age groups, the one knowing it as the stage show of 1903, the other as the film of a later era); Ivor Novello's 'Perchance to Dream' and other musicals; Noel Coward's music, especially that from 'Cavalcade'; and Herbert's 'Bless the Bride'. The suggestions given here are not by any means exhaustive, and would not be sufficient to maintain a full program of activity for any length of time, (although it will be found that considerable repetition of work is enjoyed, so that it is not necessary or even desirable to prepare an entirely new program each week). However, it will be found that after a while, as one gains experience and confidence, planning social music programs is not difficult;

patients participate more and more in their own group work, planning things for themselves, bringing records and books of music, suggesting songs, and generally participating with the minimum of direction.

Suggested song books: 'Grandma's Songs', 'Grandpa's Songs', 'Songs of the Wide World', 'Songs for Everyone', (all Australian publications, by Allans). Moody and Sankey's Hymns can sometimes be found in second-hand music shops (or even 'white elephant' stalls at church fetes), as also can old sheet music, collected volumes of ballads and religious songs. Many of these, such as 'The Lost Chord', 'The Holy City', 'The Rough Wooden Cross', 'The Stranger of Galilee', are still in print, and some of these are to be found in the volumes listed above.

Selections from musical shows: Simplified versions are available for many Gilbert and Sullivan operas. Also 'My Fair Lady', 'The King and I', 'The Sound of Music', 'Porgy and Bess', 'Kiss me Kate', 'Oklahoma', 'Show Boat', 'South Pacific', 'Carousel', all costing about 60 cents (Aust.), 20 New Pence (U.K.).

'Easy to listen to' classics: The perennial favourite, Beethoven's 'Fur Elise' is often requested, as are his so-called 'Moonlight Sonata', 'Pathetique Sonata' and the 'Minuet in G', which so many people have played in early piano lessons. Collections of favourite pieces of various composers, in the moderately difficult range, are published by Keith Prowse of London, under the general title of The Home Series of Great Masters, and these are available in many parts of the world. Each volume is devoted to the works of one of 12 composers, including Bach, Brahms, Liszt, Handel, Tchaikovsky, Mendelssohn, Schubert and Chopin.

If it is possible to obtain records, there are many collections of suitable music available. Several of the albums put out by the 'Reader's Digest' are helpful in geriatric work, as also are the sing-along records made by Mitch Miller. Re-issues of old records with the songs of Paul Robeson, John McCormack, Kenneth McKellar and others are always well received, as are discs of Scottish pipe bands (in moderation) and 'old time' dances—which will set patients' toes tapping as well as tongues wagging!

One item of equipment which would be valuable for a geriatric unit is a player-piano, or pianola, as it is often called. This enables a musical program to be arranged even if no pianist is available. Rolls of modern songs are still being made, and old rolls can often be found in second-hand shops. An interesting paragraph in a local paper would probably produce a sizable harvest of old pianola rolls, so that gradually a library of music could be built up. The activity of using a pianola would also be of physical benefit to many patients.

The form a musical social program takes naturally depends on the staff and talents available, but one should never despair of getting help from the community in this regard. Indeed, to enlist the services of a person outside the hospital as an accompanist could well help to bring the activities of a geriatric unit before a wider public. The mouth organ, the piano accordion, the guitar, and the auto-harp are all instruments which can be used as the centre of a sing-song, and these have some advantages over the more usual piano accompaniment in that the accompanist is facing the group instead of sitting either with his back to the group, or, at best, sitting twisted round—a posture which is restful for neither the performer nor the 'audience'. (The auto-harp is a simple table-top instrument which can be played merely by numbers, or can be used with normal musical notation. Teachers working with sub-normal children in the Queensland Education Department have taught themselves to use this instrument with great benefit to their pupils, as also have music therapists in other parts of the world. The cost is not high and the instrument comes in various sizes.)

Some migrants never fully settle into their new country, and if, in old age, illness separates them from family support, their plight is the worse. They may be helped by using songs from their native lands as part of a music program. This may stimulate discussion about their problems as well as providing comfort. The author has found it helpful to concentrate on music which is common to several groups (such as 'Santa Lucia', which can be sung in Italian or in English) thus providing a link between nationalities.

The most important items of equipment for any hospital musician are *imagination*, to think in terms of the patients and to use unlikely material for therapeutic ends; *courage* in innovating, thinking creatively even if others say, 'You can't do it and it wouldn't be any use even if you could'; and *persistence*, to keep at it even if one meets with apathy or active discouragement.

11. *Discussion group work*

As has already been described, music can be used to set the scene for therapeutic discussion work in a group, its quality of emotion being employed to create a climate conducive to the thinking-through of topics relevant to the lives of the elderly and disabled.

One of the matters which must be decided is how far the leader of the group should manipulate the discussion. Today manipulation has unpleasant overtones, suggesting intrigue and brain-washing, and the manipulative person is regarded as untrust-worthy because he twists circumstances and people for his own ends. But in a therapeutic setting, a certain amount of manipulation is necessary, even if only to make a patient feel hopeful about the outcome of treatment, or to set up conditions which will help patients to talk things over readily.

In formal psychoanalytic discussion and consultation, the therapist adopts one of several schools of thought and technique. Although there are numerous systems, most of them fall into one of two categories, that of *insight* (in which a cure for the patient's emotional disability is, it is hoped, achieved by giving him insight into his problems and the reasons which underly them, in the belief that such knowledge will enable him to overcome them), or the *behaviourist* type of approach, sometimes called 'action therapy'. In this the therapist adopts the point of view that many of our problems of behaviour persist long after the causes for the problems have disappeared, and that people can be enabled to lead happier lives, not by ascertaining causes, but by eliminating the symptoms which are presented.

Why should the distinction between these ideas of therapy be relevant, since we are not embarking on psychotherapy as such, but only on what might be called 'therapeutic conversation'? In all our dealings with patients, we are, whether we recognise it or not, committed to one of these two points of view. When we see a patient in a state of distress, we may either adopt a 'Cheer up' actionist approach—i.e. dealing with the *symptoms* of grief—or we may adopt the 'Find out why' approach, trying to sort out the *reasons* and, if possible, deal with them (i.e. the insight approach). Because of circumstances, we may even follow each method in turn, first cheering the patient at a superficial level, and later, at what may be a more appropriate time, dealing with the causes.

This leads on to another of the major difficulties in talking with patients about their problems—namely, how far one's own point of view, one's ethical and moral standard, affects the discussion. This may not be as major a problem in the work of a geriatric unit as in a unit for psychiatric patients, or for perplexed younger adults, but nevertheless ethical and moral queries do arise. As was pointed out earlier, there are many marital difficulties which arise in later life, as well as other problems in which the patient says, 'I don't know what I ought to do!' As one writer expressed it, it seems illogical to encourage a patient to talk freely about everything but not to talk back to him on any topic which involves religion or morality, for example. Followers of Rogers, the German psychologist, try to overcome this by adopting what is called a 'reflective technique'. In this method, the patient's own comments are reflected back to him, not verbatim, but with sufficient difference in mode of expression for the patient to gain a fresh point of view and fresh understanding. But however hard one tries to be impersonal and uninvolved, the patient will interpret what is said in the light of his own needs.

Dr. Perry London, in his challenging book, *The Modes and Morals of Psychotherapy*,[1] discusses the difficulties of personal ethics at some length, and points out that even refusing to give an opinion on a moral issue is, in effect, a moral stand, since it leaves the client or patient free to interpret it in his own way, and in general a refusal to give any opinion is interpreted as indicating a libertarian point of view on the part of the therapist. The relevance of this matter to informal discussion work in a geriatric unit may seem remote. Nevertheless, it is a matter which everyone connected with a hospital or other therapeutic environment should think through with great sincerity and earnestness. All members of the staff of a hospital tend to be endowed, in the eyes of patients, with more than human gifts of insight and understanding, and their views are often given greater weight of authority than is justified. It is therefore important that we should decide how far we shall allow our personal opinions to influence the course of even an apparently trivial conversation on loneliness, disability, marital relationships and so on.

All of these matters and many others may come up in informal discussion work, or it may become apparent that they *need* to be brought to the surface. The social worker will be able to observe such stresses in her interviews with patients and their families, or even fleeting observations of family relationships may suffice to indicate a basic lack of empathy. For example, a middle-aged daughter may betray greater impatience with a parent with Parkinson's disease—for example, when the parent is slow to get into a car to go home—and one sees the patient's rigidity and tremor increase as the mental agitation increases. One observer of such an incident may identify with the harassed daughter, who is thinking, 'She/he is just being difficult. She/he managed perfectly all right yesterday.' Another observer may identify with the parent, feeling intolerant of the daughter's impatience, and thinking, 'Down with children!' Clearly, in this and other situations it is important that one should have understanding of one's own family relationships, since our attitudes to others are profoundly influenced by our own experiences in family life. It is for this reason that so many leaders of therapeutic teams consider it essential for staff to have group experiences and gain greater insight into their reactions to patients' behaviour and difficulties.

How can we employ music to help us in talking about patients' worries and personal difficulties, whether these have resulted from growing old as such, or from the disabilities which ageing often brings? In some geriatric departments, any discussion work is undertaken by the social work department, with proper accommodation set aside (i.e. a sitting-room environment rather than an office with the telephone as a potential interruption). In others, a clinical psychologist is available to run groups, or an occupational therapist may also carry out this work. But all of these people may be interested in a combined program of work, using music sometimes as the basis for a group discussion. In some units, however, no such specialist staff are available, and it is with this eventuality in mind that the following suggestions are offered.

In planning a directed group activity, rather than a purely social one, it is important to think well ahead, and work out possible directions of thought, preferably with two or more avenues available, since people do not react as predictably as one might imagine. Any one piece of music may lead into several different trains of thought, and spontaneity will be dulled if the leader of the group wrenches the conversation around in an attempt to follow a predetermined pattern whenever it seems that a new line of ideas is being developed. An example of how ideas are born out of music can be seen in the following:

In the 'Grand Canyon Suite', by Ferde Grofe, one piece entitled 'Sunrise' is a portrait in music of the time before dawn, the first stirrings of bird-life, and the sunrise. On one occasion, the playing of this record led into a discussion of life in the country as compared with life in the city, the peace and quiet of life away from towns, and so on. On another occasion, the same record gave rise to a tense discussion on waiting for things to happen, wondering what was to occur, fears of what might be 'around the corner' and so on, this being stimulated by the early part of the music which portrays the waiting time before the sunrise. Differences between the two discussions suggested by the same record are not always as marked as this, but one cannot plan on any precise development of conversation—although with leading questions one may in part manipulate the group so that desired topics are brought to the surface for the benefit of the patients.

The following is a list of a few records, with some questions or ideas which might be presented to lead into particular themes related to problems of ageing.

1. Strauss waltzes. Starting by conjuring up a mental picture of a ballroom scene, with the elaborate 'romantic' style of dressing (aided by pictures, if good examples are available, which can readily be seen by the whole group), the discussion may then go on to changing styles of clothes, and whether this truly indicates a change in outlook on life, or is merely a matter of superficial appearance. Do we find it hard to understand people who look very different from ourselves in their general style? Does this affect relationships between the generations?

2. 'Always' (Irving Berlin) and 'With a Little Bit of Luck' (Frederick Lowe). These two songs present contrasting views of love and marriage, and of enduring affection. Which is closer to reality? This can lead on to a profitable discussion on roles within marriage, the effects on these of ageing, retirement and disability, the balance of partnership, as well as the need to support each other when things go wrong. (This phrase is included in the words of 'Always', so the topic should arise quite naturally.)

3. Modern church music—for example Beaumont's 'Folk Mass' or similar music by Malcolm Williamson. Possible questions

which might stimulate discussion: Does the use of modern idiom in music bring the Churches into line with modern thought? Are young people more interested in membership of a church if modern music is used, e.g. the guitar Mass often held in Roman Catholic churches, and similar ideas in Church of England and Protestant churches? Do we feel that our beliefs are threatened by the use of such music because it indicates change? Can we cope with these feelings when they occur?

4. The song, 'My Old Man's a Dustman', popular in the late 1950s, is still well-known and greatly enjoyed. From it we may lead on to talk about the relative status of different types of work in the eyes of the community, feeling of inferiority when one no longer has a job, and possibly from this to feelings about retirement. (This song was on one occasion used in a different way, with a patient who was being very disruptive to a group of withdrawn psychotic patients by shouting out 'Garbage!' to every suggestion made to the group. It was suggested to him that he might enjoy singing a garbage song, and when 'My Old Man . . .' was played, he did join in, with great good humour, and ceased his previous pattern of behaviour.)

5. A song popular in the 1940s, 'Money Is the Root of All Evil', may be remembered by persons in a geriatric group, and could well be used as the peg on which to fasten a discussion about the financial needs of the elderly. This may seem a flippant approach to a problem which causes such distress to so many of the ageing, but because of its very flippancy one is more likely to penetrate to hidden feelings than when defensive mechanisms are aroused in a more serious approach.

The foregoing are but a few of the many ideas which could be followed through after playing records or singing songs, and it takes only some imaginative planning to bring to the surface any problem which is worrying patients. Then they can be helped to cope with the problem either emotionally or practically by the group's support or professional consultation.

Although not a musical stimulus, it is interesting to play a record or a tape recording of everyday sounds of traffic, shopping bustle, and so on. Formal recordings of these are available on extended play discs of moderate price—or one can take a tape recorder into the street and tape the day-by-day sounds as they occur. For patients who have been in hospital or nursing home for a long time, these sounds help to re-orientate them by bringing to mind the sounds which once were a part of their lives. It sometimes happens that the topic which such records arouse is the loss of 'alone-ness' and privacy. Although few people want to be lonely, most of us like occasionally to be alone, and for those elderly people who are in nursing homes and hospitals solitude is a forgotten luxury unless they can afford a single room.

REFERENCE

1. London, P. *The Modes and Morals of Psychotherapy*, Holt, Rinehardt and Winston, New York, 1964.

12. *Specific conditions—planning music therapy for particular purposes*

GENERAL KEEP-FIT WORK

In keep-fit work, the aim is to maintain a standard of physical fitness which is comparable with what would be expected in a person not disabled by a stroke or other condition, taking into account the unavoidable diminution of ability imposed by the disease. For example, a patient who is in a wheelchair because of a severe stroke, may also show weakness of abdominal muscles quite independently of the stroke itself, and such weakness can be mitigated by appropriate programs of exercises. The intention of a keep-fit program should be to exercise each area of the body each day, with maintenance of joint mobility and of muscle tone wherever this is not rendered impossible by organic disease.

Head and neck

This area of the body is frequently beset by stiffness and tension, leading to headaches and general muscular discomfort. Rolling movements, with suitable musical accompaniment to emphasise the smooth nature of the movement required, should be used. It will often be necessary for the patient's head to be held firmly but gently from behind to encourage the full range of movement in a smooth manner, without jerks and tension, preceded if necessary by a gentle rubbing of the neck muscles to relax the tension so often encountered here. If giddiness results from these rolling movements, even if the patient's eyes are closed, then stop the movement. Music for this should preferably have a 6/8 rhythm, which gives the necessary swinging atmosphere without briskness, and should be slow. Such pieces as 'The Skye Boat Song' are excellent—if they are played slowly and gently—or a 'dreamy' waltz tune such as 'The Skaters Waltz'. It is best if patients are allowed to work at their own pace in this type of activity, since nothing is gained by speed. Indeed, speed is often inimical to success.

Shoulders and arms

Here, there is often the problem of total or partial paralysis from a cerebrovascular accident, with the all too common painful or 'frozen' shoulder joint. Many rehabilitation experts believe that such problems are entirely avoidable if the right techniques of moving a disabled patient are employed from the outset, with correct slings to prevent stretching the joint merely by the dead-weight of a paralysed arm. However, such disabilities are en-countered, either because of bad handling or because there has been an old injury which has been aggravated by hemiplaegia. When the shoulder is completely 'frozen', the physiotherapist alone can decide what should be done—but even here, musical accompaniment to work on, say, a shoulder wheel may make the work more effective by raising pain threshold and calming fears. For patients whose shoulders are slightly stiff or tense, similar rotating movements to those described for head and neck may be used, with, where necessary, the uninvolved hand to guide a paralysed arm and shoulder.

For patients with hemiplaegia, many of whom sit all day with one shoulder higher than the other, exaggerated shrug-ging movements up to the ears and down again are helpful. For accompaniment, simple chords played on the piano are effective, moving up the keyboard to signify the upwards motion, and down the keyboard again to indicate that the shoulders are to drop back again. By improvising in this way, one can adapt the timing of the exercise to suit the circumstances. If no accompanying instrument is available, then a record can be used. Again, this should not be in any way a brisk piece of music. Something of the general mood and speed of the songs 'Santa Lucia' or 'Ra-mona' would be acceptable.

Feet and legs

Rotating of ankle joints, first in one direction and then the other is of benefit to the chairbound—especially those who, it is hoped, will become mobile again—in keeping suppleness of feet and ankles. For these exercises, it is best if patients sit temporarily with their legs crossed, in order to leave each leg in turn free from weight. But it should be emphasised to the patients that crossing the legs, whether at knee or ankle level, is an unwise procedure for any length of time, because of damage to the circulatory processes. (One need not go into details of deep-vein thrombosis, but merely say, 'It is unwise.')

In this exercise, where tension is not so frequent a problem, the music used can be of a brisker nature. 'The Merry Widow Waltz' and 'The Blue Danube' are suitable.

Toe-tapping is greatly enjoyed, and indeed many patients do this quite unwittingly when music is played. It can be employed for therapeutic ends by encouraging a heel-toe action, not just a toe-tapping with the heel resting on the ground. This action becomes still more beneficial to the leg musculature if, instead of merely pivoting to and fro from heel to toe, the leg is raised off the ground in between, making use of the quadriceps muscles. This is quite hard work, and one cannot expect patients to keep it up for long, but it is of great assistance to walking. A most suitable piece of music for this is the Scots song 'The Keel Row', not only because of its brisk swinging rhythm but also because the sound of the title is so reminiscent of the words 'heel-toe', so that one sees what is almost a proprioceptive feedback. Of benefit also is the lifting of the leg or legs, held horizontally with straight knee. In this, the hemiplaegic patient should be able to use the unaffected leg to assist the affected leg, and even if there is an additional weight of a caliper to raise, the additional muscle strengthening will be of value. (However, one should encourage the lifting of a paralysed limb without such assistance if possible.)

It will be realised that this particular exercise benefits the abdominal muscles, and at first some patients may need to hold on to the seat of the chair in order to swing the legs up, hold for a second or more before lowering. The lowering of the legs should be a controlled movement, not a flop or a crash, and is in fact harder to keep under control than the raising up because of the working against gravity. The timing of this exercise is important, and ideally the accompaniment should be improvised so that the length of the time the legs can be held horizontally can be gradually built up. A simple chord accompaniment such as was described for the shrugging of shoulders is helpful, but, if this is not possible, then the song 'Those Magnificent Men in Their Flying Machines' provides a humorous atmosphere, with the *idea* of lifting and lowering even if the timing of the song does not match the timing of the exercise.

For patients with painful knee joints, the use of a high exercise stool can be of benefit, with the legs being swung to and fro to music. As with the frozen shoulder, the function of the music is to allay fear, and thus increase the range of movement which may be obtained. The high stool is needed to ensure that the legs do not have to be held off the ground (which is a tiring procedure for any length of time), but can swing naturally. Hands and fingers should be stretched, and with a barefoot group toe stretching can be undertaken, the toes being alternately stretched out and curled under (extended and flexed). For patients who are expected to walk again, this is helpful, since toes are used in walking more than patients usually realise, unless they have been unlucky enough to lose a toe, when the realisation is forced upon them. 'My Favourite Things' from 'The Sound of Music' fits these movements.

Trunk and spine

For patients who do not suffer from ataxia or general giddiness, a movement involving curling over the whole body and then straightening up is helpful, so long as it is done slowly. The posture achieved at the end of the movement is often markedly better than the posture usually held, with benefits to respiration in particular, as well as to aching backs and shoulders. No precise timing can be suggested for such a movement; the speed will depend on the patient's individual build and temperament. However, it is helpful to have a musical background to give a purposeful atmosphere. A song such as 'The Charmaine Waltz' might be used, or, if a brisker movement is required, a march tune could be played.

Another exercise of benefit to the trunk but with no prohibitions for ataxic patients is the general tightening of muscles achieved by holding the tummy in and pushing back against the back of the chair at the same time, holding this position for a moment before relaxing. 'Come to the Fair' would be a suitable tune for such an exercise, the length of time the held-in position is maintained being varied at will for different numbers of lines of the song.

The time which the total program should occupy will be determined by the physical condition of the group of patients concerned. No firm ideas on this can be given, except to say that the aim should be to increase the time and difficulty of the program in order to build up tolerance to exercise and capacity for muscular activity. In this aim, the 5BX plan of exercises makes helpful reading, although the plan of work laid down would be inappropriate for the geriatric group catered for here.

Records with pamphlets on keep-fit exercises are available under several manufacturers' labels. They are usually classified as 'music and movement', and although the exercises themselves would in general be unsuitable for elderly patients, the accompaniment could be used for many of the exercises suggested above.

MUSIC THERAPY IN DISUSE SYNDROMES

Mention has already been made of decubitus ulcers as a disuse problem in which music would assist by increasing general alertness and level of activity, since it has been demonstrated that there is an inverse correlation between the incidence of pressure sores and the number of spontaneous movements which a patient makes.

Contractures developed by apathetic patients are another disuse syndrome in which musical activity might have a role to play by increasing a patient's mobility and range of movement. In a psychogeriatric group, there are many movements which can be incorporated into action songs and games, as what might be called 'hidden physiotherapy'. Such activities are:

1. 'Rock My Soul in the Bosom of Abraham', clapping and using arm movements for 'so high, so wide' etc. Apart from its good effects on muscles, it helps those who may have developed nihilistic tendencies, because it stresses the existence and position of parts of the body. The same is true of any action song which names parts of the body.

2. 'Inceywincey Spider' appears to the middle-aged or young to be so much a kindergarten song as to be ludicrous, but it is acceptable in a psychogeriatric group and—if carefully presented —even in an ordinary geriatric group. In this song, the hands are stretched upwards, outwards and downwards, and a good range of chest and shoulder expansion is achieved if the actions are done enthusiastically.

3. 'Little Peter Rabbit Had a Fly Upon His Nose' also emphasises the position of some parts of the body, and uses finger and arm actions.

Exton-Smith[1] mentions work done by Brocklehurst with pelvic floor exercises to reduce incontinence. If these can be explained to a group, music would provide a good basis by giving the timing of the 'holding in' of the muscles and encouraging correct performance of the exercises. Any waltz tune would be suitable, since the exact timing would be altered to increase the muscular tone over a period of time. One could start off, for example, with one bar of music for 'holding in', then one bar for relaxation, then increasing the number of bars of music in which the muscles would be held.

Hypostatic pneumonia is a disuse syndrome in which singing could be of benefit by encouraging the patient to use adequate breathing methods and also by encouraging an interest in living. The idea of singing sessions in a ward of a general hospital will, to some people, appear not only impossible but probably undesirable as well. However, if the co-operation of the nursing staff can be obtained to establish musical work on a trial temporary basis, the results will probably be so marked that the work will continue permanently. The provision of accompaniment is a problem, but even a mouth-organ is better than nothing. The guitar or piano-accordion are ideal. They are portable, and one can move from one bed to another, playing personal requests and—if necessary—avoiding those patients who for some reason should not be disturbed. It is interesting to note how sometimes patients who 'hate being disturbed and hate everything and everybody', will start to sing and say they have enjoyed the music session. If this can be done in a general hospital, in which acutely ill patients are being treated, how much more readily can it be arranged in a geriatric hospital, in which many patients are found together with similar disabilities, mainly of a chronic nature.

Mention has already been made of the assumption by some writers on rehabilitation that psychological deterioration should be classed as a disuse syndrome. To overcome this, music should be one of the avenues of activity undertaken. Long-stay patients should be encouraged to choose their own programs of music, to be played over the hospital's intercom or piped music system. (And now that the provision of piped music facilities is allowed for Australian Commonwealth subsidy under the Aged Persons' Homes Act, it is likely that more nursing homes will install such systems.) It is essential, however, if the use of such a system is to be therapeutic and not merely a sop to convention and the *appearance* of providing stimulating experiences, that it should be used intelligently. The mere playing over and over again of a few taped programs of music, with no breaks for silence, and no choice of music by patients, would not combat disuse phenomena and might indeed exacerbate these by producing an auditory shutting-out of the unwanted stimuli through sheer boredom at the same tunes being played repeatedly.

It is advisable that a good variety of music should be played, that this should not occupy all the time, and that programs should be planned by patients. It might perhaps be decided that there should be a one-hour session each morning and afternoon, apart from music used as accompaniment to programs of exercises. Exact details of this nature can only be determined by circumstances, of the age, frailty and interests of the patients concerned.

RELAXATION AND MUSIC

Tension in patients manifests itself in many ways. It may be seen in the posture which betrays a tenseness of muscles; it may be heard in a tense voice; it may be seen in sudden flashes of hostility and aggression in those who generally appear placid; it may be shown in aches and pains, especially of the head and neck. How can music help?

In a Utopian establishment, one can visualise a large number of exercise mats, on each of which lies an elderly patient, relaxing and perhaps even sleeping for a while, in a good relaxed posture. Such a situation is common enough in antenatal care, but less in geriatric work. However, it should be borne in mind as a possibility for decreasing tension. The music played should be soothing, and this is one area in which the impersonality of recorded music has a place. Patients are more likely to relax physically when they know a record will continue to the end than if they are wondering what to ask for next. The Melachrino Strings and records with such titles as 'Music for Dining' should prove suitable. The volume should be loud enough for people to hear without straining, but not so loud as to be over-stimulating, and it is for this reason that 'restaurant' music is ideal, since it is intended to provide a restful background without obtruding itself on patrons' conversations. This is the level of sound which is required for relaxation techniques. Music alone may not suffice to relax some patients; it will be necessary to show them how to let their limbs feel heavy and gradually to relax. One hospital patient expressed the wish for music at bedtime to help him relax: during the music session he found himself, to his own irritation, dropping off to sleep, when really he wanted to listen, and he then suggested that soft music at bedtime would help those who were sleepless and in pain to relax and 'drop off'.

This is another situation in which piped music would have therapeutic advantages, as long as any patient who had an antipathy to it could switch it off. We each have our tastes and preferences in music and no one piece yet composed will suit everybody, and thus it is essential to maintain the integrity of the individual by allowing him to turn the music off at will.

At a symposium given in London in 1964 under the auspices of the then Society for Music Therapy and Remedial Music (now the British Society for Music Therapy), papers were read about work being done in various hospitals in relaxation, including the use of music to assist in the relaxation of tension.[2] Although the work described was being carried out with patients in a psychiatric setting, or, as in the Uffculme clinic in Birmingham, at an out-patients clinic for the tense and anxious, much of the work is applicable to any group of patients, since any illness or disability tends to bring in its wake a certain anxiety about the future—except for those who exhibit an unreal response to the situation with euphoria or denial. Thus any group of geriatric patients is likely to benefit from sessions of listening to music in a relaxed atmosphere. The time immediately before settling down at night would be most appropriate in those hospitals equipped with facilities for piped music. In day units, or in residential units during the day, an after-lunch session would also be helpful in providing a relaxing atmosphere for quiet rest. In the U.S.A. some evidence suggests that in nursing homes where music is used in social setting there is less aggressiveness between patients.[3]

MUSIC FOR RESPIRATORY PROBLEMS

In talking and working with the elderly and disabled, one realises that many of them have little concept of the mechanisms of breathing. This is probably true for the majority of people—for example, we are usually aware of the diaphragm only when suffering from hiccups. However, when we are considering the disabled—many of whom spend the greater part of life either sitting or lying—this unawareness has disadvantages. One sees that many patients are using only the apex of the lungs, and indeed think of the lungs as being in the region of the shoulders and sternum, so that there is restricted exchange of air in respiration. Frequently the air at the base of the lungs remains static.

For some patients, there is a need for specific work in breathing techniques. This will generally be carried out under the guidance of a physiotherapist, patients continuing their work between visits of, or to, the therapist. For some in small nursing homes, however, constant physiotherapy may not be feasible, and the following suggestions are given for general breathing exercises which should be beneficial, the musical accompaniment giving added interest and enjoyment to the work, and, for such conditions as emphysema, the necessary rhythm.

It is helpful to start with a brief discussion of the extent of the lungs, perhaps making use of clear illustrations or such figures as 'The transparent man', with removable parts to show the relative positions of various organs. This will give a feeling of how large the lungs are, how the diaphragm lies across the body, and so on. One can then go on to point out the types of breathing used, with the emphasis on intercostal muscles (which can, for simplicity, be referred to as 'rib muscles') , diaphragm and abdominal muscles. Some find it hard to comprehend abdominal breathing, but getting them to take notice of *how* they are breathing when they wake in the mornings will make them aware that they do in fact use abdominal techniques. One can help patients to realise where the diaphragm is by reminding them of what happens when they have hiccups, as well as by showing a picture or figure. The intercostal muscles present little difficulty in recognition; it is easy to place the hands on the lower part of the rib cage and feel the expansion taking place as one breathes in.

It is often observed that those who organise breathing exercises start the cycle by asking patients to breathe *in*. It is, however, more satisfactory to ask them first to breathe right out, with hands on ribs to help push the air out, and even to ask them to 'make their lungs whistle', so that they can feel the full extent of the lungs and empty out all the 'old air'. (This should be presented as a light-hearted proceeding, not because it is unimportant from a therapeutic point of view, but in order to gain maximum co-operation in a cheerful atmosphere. Some patients are prone to take umbrage at the implied suggestion that they do not know how to do something as simple as breathing!) From a physiological point of view the 'breathing out to start' principle is sound, since the cycle of inspiration and expiration is triggered by *lack* of oxygen and the need to refill the lungs, not by having full lungs and the need to expel air. One therefore starts all breathing exercises by exhaling, and then going on to inhaling. By exhaling first, one also avoids air trapping.

Breathing in through the nose is to be encouraged, since the nose acts as a filter, and generally one breathes out through the mouth. The exact timing depends on the condition of the patients, the more frail being unable to sustain such a long cycle, and those with emphysema, or similar obstructive conditions, need to lengthen the breathing out part of the cycle compared with the

G

breathing in part. However, for general purposes, a pattern of not more than five deep breaths, three seconds expiration followed by three seconds inspiration is satisfactory. Suitable music for this would be either a very slow waltz, played with a metronome setting of 60, or a piece with the time signature of 9/8, metronome setting of $\bullet$. = 60 would give a suitable flowing feeling to the work.

It is recommended that for emphysema, the correct timing for breathing should be $1\frac{1}{2}$ seconds inspiration, $\frac{1}{2}$ second pause, three seconds expiration.[4] Since this would entail music in a rhythm of 5, choice of accompaniment is limited, but the wellknown theme from Tchaikovsky's 'Pathetique' Symphony in 5/4 time could be used. The reason for the prolonging of the expiratory phase is that a major problem in this disease is the trapping of air, and by prolonging the breathing out there is more chance of expelling air. Patients usually find that it is helpful to purse the lips in breathing out. Blocker and Gonzalez[5] recommend that for all chronic pulmonary obstructive diseases exercises should be used which will improve and co-ordinate muscles of respiration. They say that exhaling should take exactly twice as long as inhaling (whether for emphysema, chronic bronchitis, asthma, bronchiolitis, fibrosa obliterans, bronchiolectasis, or a combination of these). Providing musical accompaniment for this 2:1 ratio is easier than for the 2:3 system mentioned above, since any piece of music will do, patients using one bar of music to breathe in and two bars to breathe out. Avoid, however, a piece such as 'The Blue Danube', which is written strongly in a four-bar pattern, unless the patients can sustain a pattern of one bar inhaling followed by three bars exhaling. If possible, the most satisfactory solution is to play a simple line of chords on the piano, which can be speeded up or adapted at will. These are not difficult to work out, even for those whose knowledge of written music is nil. A suitable progression would be to use middle C as the thumb note for the right hand, the middle finger on the next-but-one note (E), and the little finger on the next-but-one note to that (G). Put the left hand on a C further down the piano and play all the notes together firmly. For the next chord, move the thumb of the right hand to the note previously played by the little finger (G) and put the other fingers in the same spacing apart as before, with the left hand playing a G in the bass. This progression of two chords can be repeated up and down the piano, using the pedal to join up the sounds. As one becomes more confident, it will be found that other chords can be used to make the sound more interesting. One should never be afraid to experiment with the keyboard in private, to learn how different chords and notes produce different effects.

Assuming that the group of patients is seated, one way of assisting abdominal expulsion of air is to get them to fold the arms across, below the level of the umbilicus, and lean forwards firmly, so that the folded arms help to push the air out. One can also ask patients to place the finger tips together just below the sternum and observe how the tips separate as the lungs fill, showing that the lower parts of the lungs have been used. All of these techniques, and others which will be improvised as a need arises, will help patients to realise where their lungs are, which muscles are used in breathing, and give them a feeling for the basic principles of respiration.

In diseases such as asthma, where emotion can play such a decisive part in the progress of the condition, it is found that playing a musical instrument is beneficial. This may not be a practical proposition for many of the elderly, whose financial resources and deficiencies of both vision and hand function prevent it. However, singing presents no such difficulties, and in the enjoyment of a pleasant group activity the patient often forgets to worry about his breathing and the problem of 'getting rid' of air, thus achieving good ventilation and avoiding air trapping. (With children, the playing of recorders is frequently used for this purpose.)

Thus music may be used in two ways in a program designed to improve ventilation—it may be employed to give rhythm and added enjoyment to the performance of routine exercises; it may also be used in singing for what might be termed 'disguised therapy', particularly in those diseases in which there is an element of the psychosomatic.

By improving respiration, we improve the patients' tolerance to activity, and thus break through the vicious cycle of anoxia and dyspnoea/reduced activity/muscular atrophy and weakness/apathy in environment/depression which is seen in those suffering from chronic pulmonary disease, and, to a lesser degree, in all those whose way of life, imposed by disability, is sedentary.

MUSIC FOR CO-ORDINATION AND REBUILDING PROPRIOCEPTION

As the result of different lesions in the central nervous system, patients will be found to suffer from different forms and different degrees of inco-ordination and unawareness of position in personal and extra-personal space. Many of these are associated with lesions in what is usually defined as the parietal lobe of the brain, although as Critchley[6] points out this area of the brain has no clear physiological boundaries, and its separation from the rest of the brain is largely a matter of convention. However, it is observed that damage to the parietal area of the brain does result in some disorientation and unawareness of position or even unawareness of the existence of parts of the body (agnosia), difficulties in carrying out actions (apraxia), and other associated phenomena. Frequently these are found in conjunction with speech difficulties, either involving thought processes (aphasia or dysphasia), or articulation (anarthria and dysarthria). However, some lesions of the parietal lobe cause agnosia without speech pathology, and in this case the problems may at first escape detection.[7, 8] It is therefore necessary for a music therapist to be on the lookout for problems of position in space, etc., particularly of left and right, since these often show up in musical activities, in which actions are keyed to words of a song. (Many patients suffering from these disabilities were unaware of the fact until told by a neurologist.[9]) With any patient who has been regarded as obstinate or unco-operative, we must be on the *qui vive* for agnosia, since it has been suggested, with good evidence to support the idea, that many patients who appear obstinate or apathetic about recovery from a stroke are in fact suffering from agnosia, and do not realise that the affected side belongs to them, bizarre as this may appear.[10]

For patients in whom problems of proprioception have been detected, music offers some hope. Descriptions have been given earlier as to how one may approach these problems. More detailed suggestions follow: Draw an outline of the patient's two hands on the table or a board, bigger than life size, the degree of enlargement depending on the degree of inco-ordination, so that for a patient who is only mildly affected, the 'hand' drawn is only a little larger than his own, but for a severely incoordinated patient, a very large hand is drawn. Working with a slow march tune, the patient then places his hands down on the table, trying to fit within the outline, and either saying 'left right' as he does it, or—if he cannot speak—listening to someone saying these words clearly as he moves his hands. As placing improves, the size of the hand outline drawn is decreased. 'Left' and 'right' should be marked on the patient's hands so that conditioning is through **visual** as well as tactile and auditory modes.

Similar techniques should be adopted with the placing of the feet, with outlines drawn on the floor or on a board. The accompaniment should also be gradually speeded up, not to the extent of producing mental tension, but almost imperceptibly, to give a quicker response.

Using cymbals of different sizes, the patient can also learn to distinguish three-dimensional space. At first, large cymbals are used, so that the problem of producing a sound by striking the two together is only slight, since there is a large degree of leeway in the accuracy required of placing the cymbals for them to touch each other. The size of cymbals chosen is then decreased, until one is using the tiny finger cymbals, which require a fairly accurate placing for the edges to be struck together and a sound produced. In that the sound thus made is pleasant, it is a psychological reinforcement as well as an auditory stimulus to the brain indicating that co-ordination has been successful.

Rhythm sticks can be used in a similar manner, with bands of colour which must be matched up as the sticks are struck together. The width of the band of colour can be reduced until accurate placement is achieved. This is a less satisfactory method from a learning point of view, since, unlike the cymbal technique, a mis-hit (unless one misses altogether) still produces a sound from the sticks, even if one does not strike the desired colour band. However, it is a cheap and easy technique, since lengths of wooden dowelling are almost negligible in cost whereas cymbals are more costly.

With these methods, the brain is educated via a three-fold pathway—with a tactile stimulus (in the feeling of the hands), with a visual stimulus (in how the hands, or feet, look when they are correctly placed), and in the auditory stimulus (either in the sound of the voice saying 'left, right' or the sound of the musical instrument).

In agnosia, rather similar techniques may be adopted. In problems of left and right (somatolateral agnosia), tapping of the feet, while marching music is played and the words 'left, right' are said, is as effective as any. Do not employ any movement of the hands at the same time. The patterning of body movements is such that one uses the right hand, swinging to and fro, as one uses the left foot. Although people in normal health can deliberately match up right hand with right foot, the natural tendency when walking is to swing right hand with left foot, and even in a seated position, there is a *feeling* of this diagonal matching of limbs. This may be merely a subjective phenomenon, but there is no point in muddling people.

In Gerstmann's syndrome, there will be seen finger agnosia, in which patients cannot distinguish one finger from the other when the two hands are laced together, and, in some cases, cannot distinguish their own fingers from those of another in this position. This agnosia, being invariably allied with an inability to work with numbers, is a most disabling symptom of this particular form of brain damage.[8, 10] Insofar as it admits of improvement (i.e. when it is the result of a once-only trauma, or cerebrovascular accident, and not the result of an encroaching neoplasm), it too may sometimes be helped by retraining. The author has had some success with the use of musical stimuli. (So far there is no statistical evidence to support this claim since the number of cases treated is not sufficient to permit formulation of an hypothesis, and it may well be that recovery would have taken place anyway. However, the methods employed are presented here as being worth trying for any patient who has agnosia of this type.)

The patients hold up the right hand first, opposing the fingers to the thumb in turn, thus making a circle, while saying, 'Right index, right middle, right ring finger, right little finger', fitting this to a musical accompaniment of strong four-count metre. Similarly with the left hand. (The music must be slow enough to permit these actions to be done without haste; one movement to each bar of march rhythm would be suitable.) Similar actions may be performed to music—touching, for example, the right ear, the right eye, then left ear and left eye. The music serves to give a rhythm, not speed, to the movement.

For patients who have in general become unaware either of where various parts of the body are in space, or of the names of the parts of the body, one action song has been very successful. It is sung to the tune 'There Is a Tavern in the Town', and the words are:

> Head, shoulders, knees and toes, knees and toes,
> Head, shoulders, knees and toes, knees and toes, and
> Eyes and ears and mouth and nose,
> Head, shoulders, knees and toes, knees and toes.

This is not as gymnastic an operation as it might appear. It can be done well by seated patients, and it is not essential that the toes should actually be touched for the song to be effective, so long as the patient *looks* at and points to them while singing the appropriate lines of the song. One patient who suffered from both an expressive and receptive aphasia learnt to sing this song and to point to the named parts of the body even though his speech remained limited to some stereotyped phrases such as 'I don't know', and, until learning this song, his idea of the parts of the body was very vague.

Other songs can be made up to suit the needs of particular patients. The 'Hokey Pokey'—with the sections 'You put your *right* foot in' and 'You put your *left* foot in'—can also be done when patients are chair-fast, except for the verse 'You put your whole self in'. The line '. . . turn around' can be altered either to 'wave around', in which case a circle is drawn in the air, or 'look around', in which the head is turned from side to side. Either of these actions is of therapeutic benefit, for rotating the shoulders and loosening neck muscles respectively. When improvising similar songs, choose music which is so well known as to need no effort, so that concentrated thought is confined to actions. For example, one might take the tune of 'Clementine' and put the words (with appropriate actions) of

> Point the *right* hand
> Then the *left* hand,
> And the *right* hand
> Then the *left*,
> Stamp the *right* foot etc.

The timing of this is good, in that it is unhurried, so that those who have to think hard as to which side is which are not flustered by speed, but as the actions become more confident the song can be speeded up a little. Other well-known tunes can be used in a similar way. Never confuse a patient by standing opposite him to show left and right, always stand *next* to him.

In all these 'classic conditioning' techniques, the external stimulus is gradually withdrawn.

MUSIC FOR REHABILITATION AFTER BRAIN DAMAGE,
ESPECIALLY STROKE

In the re-orientation and comforting of those who are confused and disorientated after brain damage, music played quietly without any attempt at patient-participation is helpful. It should be music with which the patient is likely to be familiar, and it is worth asking relatives whether the patient has any favourite songs, since these will be especially helpful. To decide what type of music to play, check on the patient's background as well as his age—whether he is an old soldier, for example, or whether hymns are likely to be well-known. Sometimes it is necessary to go right back in time to childhood, playing Sunday School songs or even nursery tunes, in the quest for familiarity. As the acute phase passes, it is observed that the patient will join in a song, even though he shows no other sign of mentation, and gradually, in cases which are going to improve, the degree of participation increases.

After brain damage from such trauma as road accidents, one notices that the patient usually cannot control his singing to match the speed of either the accompaniment or the rest of the group. This is probably related to the emotional instability seen in such head injuries. It sometimes proves to be an indicator of general improvement when the patient starts to sing with the rest of the group, in time with the accompaniment.

The instrument which should be used in the early stages of brain damage must, of necessity, be a portable one. The patient will be in a ward, where it is improbable that a piano will be found, and in any case it is important to make personal contact with the patient, playing specifically to him, and the piano is a rather impersonal instrument unless the two people can sit virtually side by side, one playing and the other listening. It is advisable, therefore, to use a guitar, autoharp, piano accordion, transistorised chord organ of a table-top type, or a small folding harmonium of the type which used to be called a 'camp organ'. Any of these can be taken directly to the patient's bedside and played quietly to him.

As the patient's condition starts to improve, it will be seen in all probability that, when the music begins, his posture changes; he will adopt a more upright sitting position, and may turn his head towards the music even when in general his head is turned away from the involved side, and the music is played on the involved side. (It is a good general rule to play music, or indeed carry out any activity, on the uninvolved side within the line of vision, but it is also helpful to ascertain whether the patient is able to turn the head in the other direction by (for a few moments only) playing to him from the involved side.)

As the patient's condition improves to the extent of his taking part in group activities, other musical stimuli can be used. If he can speak he will, of course, be able to ask for his favourite tunes to be played. If, however, he cannot speak, suggest songs which he is likely to know, such as were played earlier in the ward situation, and encourage him to signify in some way or another his reaction to these. Despite aphasia he may even be able to sing,[11] and this is encouraging for the patient. Communication is so vital to our existence that even if it consists only of nods, frowns, or smiles of assent, we shall have achieved something in this vital area.

The boundary between social and therapeutic activity is almost indefinable. A gay polka will set our feet tapping, and this can merge imperceptibly into an exercise to strengthen quadriceps muscles and 'hamstrings'. A well-known song sets us humming the melody, and this becomes a way of improving breathing. A stirring march makes us more alert, we sit up—and our whole posture improves thereby, with many physical benefits.

Percussion band gives another example of this double purpose. It can be seen simply as fun (and the lives of most of the elderly are lamentably deficient in fun), and it can also have a therapeutic purpose. By presenting band work as an adult activity, pointing out and demonstrating by records that it is one section of a full symphony orchestra (and the only one in which we can all participate without having to acquire elaborate techniques), band work will prove acceptable to all but the most 'difficult' patients.

Sleigh bells on an oval handle can be slipped over the knuckles of paralysed hands, and either moved passively by the uninvolved hand or by even minor movements of the involved limb. Such bells are so responsive that even a small shoulder movement will make them ring, showing the patient that his efforts have been successful and also indicating audibly the position in space of the hand and arm. This sounding of the bells by a hand which has been thought of by the patient as totally incapacitated is good for the morale, and is likely to lead to renewed efforts in general physiotherapy.

As hand function returns, the instrument should be changed to a castanet or a bell on a straight handle, the handle being built up with foam plastic to sufficient diameter for the patient to hold with minimum effort. Gradually the layers of padding are removed until the normal handle can be held. Later, when hand function is fairly well established, a new type of instrument altogether should be employed. This is a castanet, which resembles a half-open oyster. The two halves are joined together by an elastic band, so that a certain amount of effort is needed to close the two halves and produce a 'clack', and the elastic then opens the halves out again after the pressure is relaxed. Most of these instruments are made with a dimple on each side, and patients can thus readily use one finger at a time, opposing each in turn to the thumb. If it is felt there is too much emphasis on flexion of the hand and that the extensors are significantly weaker than the flexors, such tendencies can be counteracted by the use of bongo drums, tambourines or home-made drums, the patient tapping out rhythms with flat, horizontal fingers, or as close an approximation to this position as is possible. Such rhythmic work is also helpful to some sufferers from rheumatoid arthritis, for whom it is important that we should not exacerbate any claw-like deformity of the hand. (Such action is not possible when this deformity is already well established.)

Finger cymbals, held on the fingers by light rubber bands, and not as conventional cymbals, can be used in these circumstances also. The hands are held horizontally over a table and the cymbals tapped on the surface of the table by gentle straight-finger action. The use of cymbals for problems of co-ordination has already been described.

For patients with a muscular weakness in the forearm, making it difficult to manage alternate pronation and supination of the arm, bells on stick handles have proved useful. The instrument is very light so that no significant burden is added to the arm, and the twisting of the arm to and fro produces a pleasant sound, which acts as reinforcement to the learning process. At first it can be assisted by the uninvolved hand, but the patient should be encouraged gradually to use the involved hand and arm independently.

In assisting exercises, work with pulleys and bicycle devices can be made more interesting with musical accompaniment, the rhythm of the music aiding performance. Choose a lively tune such as a polka, which will have a steady beat. (Old time dances are all suitable.) Several exercises are helpful in hemiplaegia, apart from those done in the course of treatment by a physio-therapist, and these can well be done in a group with musical accompaniment.

1. For hand function: Stretch the hand open ('like a starfish' is a good description of the movement required), then close to a tight fist. A tune such as 'Phil the Fluter's Ball' is excellent for this, as also are square dances. The uninvolved hand may be used to assist in this action.

2. Heel and toe tapping has already been mentioned. Percy Grainger's 'Country Gardens' is a good tune for this.

3. For twisting the forearm: Lay the forearm across the lap, the hand palm downwards on the thigh. Lift the hand so that the index finger touches the nose. This is done rhythmically, slowly at first, with the speed increased as the action becomes more certain.

4. The involved arm is lifted up, above the head if possible. The uninvolved hand may be used to assist. The music used should be a swinging type of tune, such as the 'Skye Boat Song', using one bar for the upwards stretch and one bar for the downward swing, not attempting to fit the whole movement into one bar. (This tune can also be used for the preceding movement.)

5. Ankle rotation and wrist rotation are both helpful in maintaining mobility of the joints, and can be performed to music of a waltz type. For patients whose postural sense has been impaired by a stroke, the work described earlier for re-education in perception should be followed.

6. 'Stand-up' exercises (in which patients sit with hands on a bar, and rise to their feet, repeating this a number of times), are recommended for stroke patients.[12] They stand without *pulling* themselves upright; the bar is used for balance only. This exercise could be assisted by a musical accompaniment to encourage patients to sit down in a controlled manner, not 'flop' down.

In all therapy after brain damage, it is important not to over-stress the recovery of function, as this can prove very depressing for those who do not recover function,[13] but it is also important not to adopt a mere *laissez faire* doctrine, since function is more likely to return after re-educative therapy than if the paralysed parts of the body are left to themselves.[14, 15] One must achieve a balance in this, of strengthening the uninvolved parts to compensate for function which may prove to be permanently impaired, and of working at impaired parts to aid such recovery of function as may prove possible.

For patients with speech problems, whether these are a matter of inability to pronounce words correctly (dysarthria) or inability either to understand speech or to formulate ideas and the speech itself (differing types of aphasia), there are some aspects of music which will prove helpful. The speech therapist in charge of the case should be consulted, and she may be able to suggest ideas— for example, exercises to strengthen the muscles of speech, to stretch and work neck muscles and those of lips, tongue and areas around the mouth, and the jaw (chewing movements are helpful). For those who are utterly without speech, one of the most frightening and frustrating aspects for the patient is the inability to control the environment, and in music we may be able to rebuild the simple 'yes/no' communication, even if this is only by means of a nod or shake of the head. We can achieve this by asking, not 'What song would you like?', since, for an aphasic, no answer is possible, but 'Would you like so-and-so?'—suggesting a song which is likely to be familiar (deciding this on the basis of the patient's age and general background). The patient can then nod or shake the head, and feel that in at least one aspect of life he is making a decision. Trivial as this may seem, it is of psychological and emotional benefit. As described, some aphasiacs are able to sing. This phenomenon can sometimes be used to re-establish spontaneous speech and is, in any case, of great psychological value.

One of the most disconcerting forms of aphasia for the onlooker, and (when the patient is aware of his speech, for him also), is the inappropriate response, in which, for example, when the patient wants to express the affirmative, he actually says 'no' and vice versa. Sometimes, however, the patient's facial expression or other 'body language' makes it clear which he wishes to express, and this is seen in musical work, when one can often tell whether a song is familiar or not by the patient's body language. One may be able to make use of this to rebuild the correct use of 'yes' and 'no', and although this might appear a hopelessly restricted vocabulary, it has enabled many people to exercise significant control over their environment.

The method employed is as follows: When the patient's behaviour makes it unequivocally clear that he is feeling affirmation, one stands in front of him, nodding one's head and saying 'Yes, you know that song', or whatever simple remark is appropriate, and the patient will probably copy both word and action (echolalia and echopraxia), so that he is saying 'yes', nodding the head and *feeling* 'yes' at the same time. (Similarly, in situations in which the patient is feeling 'no', one shakes the head and says 'no' to him). Thus one may be able to rebuild the correct use of 'yes' and 'no' by conditioning.

For a patient who has been adept at playing a musical instrument, hemiplaegia can be a most distressing condition. Some pianists may be able to reconcile themselves to being one-handed pianists, and trumpet players may be able to manage to play since the trumpet is basically a one-handed instrument. For string players, however, as for performers on other two-handed instruments, the chances of playing again are remote, except when shoulder and elbow mobility are unimpaired, in which case it may be possible to strap the violin bow (or the slide of a trombone) to the involved hand, as is done for amputees, and use the uninvolved hand to play the notes.

For pianists who can accept playing with one hand alone, and are intellectually capable of reading music, there are many books of simple duets, in which the 'pupil's' part can be played by an adult with one hand only, who can thus gain satisfaction in making music with a friend or relative. There are also available pieces of music written for one hand alone, and any good music shop would be able to give advice as to what is available in this medium, and its degree of difficulty. The music therapist can also re-arrange music for patients, providing for both remaining skills and therapeutic possibilities. (This can be done for all disabled patients, not only those recovering from brain damage.)

Although there is a condition called amusia, in which the locality of the lesion prevents the patient from recognising music, Luria (describing a pianist patient at the Bordenko Institute, Moscow) has pointed out that brain damage *per se* does not preclude brilliant performance (BBC TV film, *The Mind of Man*, 1970). He also described a composer patient who, it is said, wrote his best works after a brain injury had resulted in aphasia (quoted by Hurwitz in *Gerontologia Clinica*, vol. 13, no. 5, 1970).

MUSIC THERAPY FOR DEGENERATIVE NEUROLOGICAL CONDITIONS
Multiple sclerosis

In multiple sclerosis, the presentation of the symptoms of the disease is so varied that treatment must be tailored to suit the needs of each patient. Many patients with this disease are treated by the proprioceptive neuromuscular facilitation methods mentioned earlier. Some therapists do not use these techniques, for various reasons which are outside the scope of this book. However, whatever system of treatment is adopted, one feature of the condition which music can aid in any circumstances is breathing. For those whose diaphragm is affected by multiple sclerosis, difficulties with breathing cause complications in respiratory infections, and one sees the fear-tension syndrome exacerbating the difficulties. Indeed, some of those who work with multiple sclerosis patients believe that tension is a significant feature of the condition. Music, either as a listening activity or as group singing, is of obvious benefit. One sometimes finds a patient whose voice is almost inaudible in ordinary speech—with the nasal, rather breathy quality which results from paralysis of the soft palate and other speech mechanisms—singing with a tone sufficiently firm for other members of the group to learn a new song from the patient! The psychological effects of this can be imagined. The way of helping multiple sclerosis patients to join in such an activity is at first to invite him merely to listen to others singing (assuming that the group is sufficiently heterogeneous for there to be some members for whom singing presents no difficulty). Next, one invites suggestions for favourite songs, then—with a little encouragement—the patient can usually be persuaded to join in in an undertone, until finally he is joining in on equal terms with others. After this activity has become well established, one can go on to breathing work alone, with the knowledge for both patient and therapist that breathing has been successful in the singing. With the memory of this to back up the work, one should be able to help the patient to greater reserves of air and general respiratory resources.

Proprioceptive neuromuscular facilitation techniques depend very much on the use of audible stimuli to 'trigger' the movements required. On entering a unit in which P.N.F. is used, one hears ringing through the air, 'Now pull, now pull, now pull', or other similar commands. Stimulation is also achieved through tactile pathways to the brain, in touching the part of the body which is to be used in such a way as to facilitate its correct use in the therapy. The author believes that in P.N.F. it should be possible to employ musical, rhythmical stimuli to enhance the other stimuli being used in building up the neuromuscular resources which are left intact. This is analogous to the work described earlier in the use of musical stimuli in rebuilding proprioception in perceptual defects.

Patients who lack co-ordination and who therefore walk unsteadily may be helped by music, which gives rhythm to their movements. The comments of one patient for whom a program was evolved are revealing, as backing up what was observed by physiotherapists: 'The music helps me to swing along. I feel much steadier, and I can do it away from the Centre, because no-one is going to look at you twice if you sing a song as you walk.' Two patterns were chosen, one a brisk, purposeful walk to be done to a march tune, the other a stroll, for which the patient hummed a waltz tune to himself. His comments bring out three important points. One concerns the transfer of training from clinic to home situation; he could see that by using musical stimulation he would be able readily to transfer the techniques learned at the clinic to his everyday walking. The second concerns the actual rhythmic stimulation which aided his walking; this was apparent from observation, but the patient was also subjectively aware of this. The third point is the social disadvantage under which multiple sclerosis patients find themselves; they feel self-conscious about their symptoms, especially when these include unsteadiness. Indeed, they are often suspected of being drunk. The patient felt that by using music to help his walking he would be less conspicuous than formerly, by modifying his ataxia.

As a socialising stimulus, music has a part to play in the lives of patients suffering from degenerative neurological diseases. As the disease affects the way of life more severely, music remains an enjoyable group activity, even if the activity consits only of listening to records in a friendly atmosphere. Unlike hemiplaegia, one has to allow for *decreasing* levels of activity, and it is most beneficial to establish some pattern of enjoyment which can continue in a modified form up to the end of life. Multiple sclerosis is said to be a disease characterised by euphoria, but this is by no means always so, and we can help to counteract depression or even despair by providing a means of social interaction which can continue despite increasing weakness and paralysis.

Huntington's chorea

The same is true in *Huntington's chorea*. In this disease, no physical or pharmacological treatment can offer any significant palliation or cure, and the patient is faced with inexorable deterioration into writhing, grimaces, helplessness and unintelligibility. Is it perhaps fortunate that so many patients become demented in the course of this disease, as one may hope that the helplessness of their condition is thus less distressing to them? But dementia does not invariably occur.[16] It is important for patients with Huntington's chorea to have social activity, which, as mentioned above, can continue to the end of life. If patients are seen only after speech has become unintelligible, the establishment of contact is fraught with difficulty, but—as with aphasic patients—one can achieve some sort of communication by asking questions and attempting to gauge whether the answer is a nod or a shake. Often the patient, even in the advanced stage of the disease, can manage a smile of sorts, and this is often used by

him as an affirmative, and a frown is used as a negative. By this
means one can find out which songs are wanted, by guessing at first
what songs will probably be known and watching carefully to see
whether the response is affirmative or negative. Having found a
few songs or pieces which the patient knows, one can then use
these to build up a relationship with him, referring to the tunes
as 'Mr. so-and-so's favourites' and encouraging other patients to
comment on them, so that the patient achieves some sort of
group relationship with others through the music. Clearly this is
a severely restricted relationship, but it is better than none at all
and it helps others to see the patient as a person, with likes and
dislikes, and with a right to free choice. Far from being bored
by weekly repetition of a small number of tunes, the patient is
gratified at having his preferences remembered. It is all too easy
for us to forget that inability to speak does not entail inability
to think and feel, and in playing loved melodies we are creating
one weapon in the armoury for the deadly fight against deper-
sonalisation of the terminal patient.

Parkinson's disease

One of the features of Parkinson's disease which can cause
misery to the patient is the change in quality of the voice; it
becomes flat and monotonous, and, since it is allied with inflexi-
bility of the facial features, gives the impression of one who has
lost interest in life and who no longer enjoys conversation or any
form of social interaction. The patient is often self-conscious
about these features of the disease, and does in fact withdraw from
relationships. The result is that the patient can become very
unhappy.

The patient may 'get stuck' with speech as he does with walking (akinesia, bradykinesia), unable to proceed at all (pathological
inertia) or repeating one syllable (perseveration). Luria describes
how retraining in terms of different musical pitch for each syllable
may, by bringing speech processes to a higher level of conscious
organisation, overcome these difficulties in cases of traumatic brain
damage.[17] The same would apply to these difficulties as experienced in Parkinson's disease.

In music, we can give the patient the opportunity of participating in a group activity in a setting in which people will be
understanding of the difficulties of speech and facial expression;
this is of psychological and supportive value. It is sometimes
observed that patients with Parkinson's disease will be able to sing

with greater inflexion of the voice than is heard in their speech. This can be used as not only a boost to the morale but as the basis for some work in improving the inflexion of the voice by encouraging the patient to breathe better (achieving better relaxation) and to think in terms of musical pitch when speaking. This does not always produce results, but the author has seen beneficial results by these means in psychiatric patients suffering from Parkinson's disease.

In all movements, the Parkinsonism patient is hampered if emotional tension supervenes, and it has been found that patients achieve more spontaneous movements when working with musical accompaniment to their physiotherapy than without this adjunct. It has been found that movements in multiple sclerosis, Parkinson's disease, and hemiplaegia were all significantly more controlled, faster and generally better, with music than without.[18]

In walking and turning, the Parkinsonism patient is incapable of making abrupt turns, but can turn in a sweeping circle only. This is hard to achieve for some patients, who find it hard to remember that they must adopt an entirely new technique in moving around. By using musical accompaniment to walking practice, we should be able to condition the patient, reinforcing the learning process with music to jog the memory about the methods to be used. They can be encouraged to hear the music in the 'mind's ear' for walking activity carried on away from the geriatric unit or the physiotherapy department, so that we get a carryover of the learning.

Some speech therapists approach the treatment of neurological conditions via breathing exercises, and if the patient is receiving speech therapy we should ascertain what techniques are being used and endeavour to find appropriate musical accompaniment to fit the exercises being carried out. For those very anxious about their breathing (and this is seen in diseases other than Parkinsonism), we see that singing provides a non-threatening situation in which breathing can be re-learnt without fear. At first, patients will not want to join in, for fear of sounding out of place, but in this a geriatric group will almost certainly prove very supportive. So many people have problems of one sort or another in speech that the anxious patient is reassured that no one will mind even if his voice does sound a little odd. The reason for the ability to sing, seen even in those whose speech is severely hampered, seems to lie in the rhythmic nature of the activity, and—in some very well-known songs—it approximates an automatic activity. Nevertheless, it is of value in keeping phonation going, in giving the patient the knowledge that his vocal chords are not utterly useless, and in enabling him to join in with the rest of the group.

In percussion band work, the patient with marked tremor will not be able to play a definite rhythmic pattern, and he should be given an instrument in which no such pattern can be attempted. A sleigh bell is good, in that it can be slipped over the knuckles and need not be grasped, and it has a continuous sound in which tremor will be made use of rather than being a nuisance.

Luria[19] describes how patients with Parkinson's disease can walk over a series of lines painted on the floor although they cannot walk on a plain surface, because the activity is brought thus under visual control and under control of complex cortical systems rather than subcortical systems. He tells how motor activities which had become impossible were linked to the semi-automatic act of blinking and then became possible. The suggestion above, of linking activities to the hearing of music, although not a perfect analogue has *some* similarities to the techniques of Luria.

The uses of music therapy in Parkinson's disease may be summarised as follows: They provide a means of social interaction in a supportive setting; they may assist the performance of some physical tasks, and provide a link between several different aspects of therapy.

REACTIVATION OF THE WITHDRAWN AND PSYCHOTIC

People who are in hospital for a long time, whether as psychiatric patients or because of a long-standing physical condition, tend to become institutionalised—that is to say, they become withdrawn, apathetic and, to a great extent, unaware of what is going on in the world. They may also become incontinent, not only because of a lesion in the anteromedial part of the frontal lobe (where injuries will produce urinary incontinence even in young patients) but also purely as the result of general mental deterioration.[20] A horrifying comparison has been drawn between the methods used for political ends by some countries in destroying the integrity of the mind, and the same 'methods' used, without any sinister intentions, by thoughtless treatment of the aged in some nursing homes. These are the inadequate provision and delay of opportunities for relief of bladder and bowel distension, the removal of personal clothing, and the damaging of self-respect. All of these can cause mental disintegration and consequent incontinence in even young political prisoners, so how much more readily will they affect the aged! We must treat the aged with respect, allowing them to grow old with dignity.

Where does music fit into this idea? Unfortunately, in the worst type of 'nursing home', so-called, no money would be spent on provision of music therapy, and unless someone is willing to give time and energy for this, no music program will be instituted. However, where care of patients and not making money is the main end, it should be possible for musical activities to be arranged. In these, whether we are dealing with frankly psychiatric or senile dementia cases, or with those who have merely become apathetic as the result of a long stay in an institution or hospital, the main methods to be employed will be the same.

The initial contact with patients must be through music which is likely to be familiar. We can thus penetrate the outer shell of indifference and gain some response. Having done this, we can go on to rebuild patients' self-respect—by asking them to choose songs or hymns; by commenting favourably on their singing; by making it clear that it is their requests for music which are of paramount importance. To be given a choice of activity can be of immeasurable value. Songs likely to be known are to be found in old song books and hymn books, some of which are still in print or have been re-issued in recent years.

Encourage movement in bed while singing is in progress, to reduce the likelihood of pressure sores and other disuse syndromes. Encourage those who are sitting in a day-room to dance, even if dancing consists only of holding hands and swinging the legs to and fro across the body. Nurses will usually help in this, providing support for patients who lack the courage or balance to stand alone or with another patient. It is beneficial for patients to dance with others as promoting social relationships.

In a psychiatric institution, where there will be other paramedical staff, one should aim to have a combined program of therapy, with the physiotherapist advising what movements are required for particular patients. The occupational therapist will also be able to join in a combined program for making simple instruments to be used by patients. But do not rely entirely on these; some instruments should be bought to provide the nucleus of a band, and these can be added to in order to build up the number of instruments available. Milk bottle tops strung on a wire coat hanger can provide good shakers, except for the deaf, who will not be able to hear the rather soft swishing sound produced. Tins filled with stones, however, are effective even for the deaf (so long as the deafness is not profound), as they can feel the rattle of the contents of the tin as well as hear it. Seal the edges well with adhesive tape to deter the curious from opening the tin to investigate the contents. Ice-cream tins can also be used, as drums can be made from them, with a piece of old inner tube for the 'skins'. Loop a string through the holes punched around the edges before doing any zig-zag stringing from top to bottom, to lessen the pull and tear on the rubber. Bells, which can usually be purchased from chain stores, can either be threaded on tapes or fastened to pieces of wooden dowelling to make sleigh bells. They can also be fixed to holes punched in the lids of ice-cream tins to make tambourines. Dowelling can be painted to make rhythm sticks, different tones being produced by pieces of wood of differing thickness. Cymbals can be made from lids, if it is possible to have slots cut carefully, with straps of leather or thick plastic stapled in position to make handles. Such simple instruments give good results in encouraging movements of hand and arms—even in the severely withdrawn, who usually do not move at all.

Although all of us pay lip service to the idea of religious freedom, our elderly people are, in general, deprived of freedom of worship because little provision is made for them to attend services.[21] This lack causes great distress to many of them, and it behoves us to do something about it if we can. Clearly, a music session must not be allowed to become a religious ceremony, because religious views vary so much from one person to another and because this is not the aim of the activity. However, patients will enjoy singing hymns, Sunday school songs or sacred songs such as 'The Holy City', and these can legitimately be considered one aspect of music therapy. We should also get in touch with local clergy if it is certain that no clergy visit the hospital or home. Busy as they are, ministers and priests are usually able to come to homes and hospitals to provide the sacraments for patients if the need is pointed out to them. This may appear to be outside the province of the music therapist's duties, but because it is so often in a musical setting that religious topics are discussed, the musician is the obvious person to make the contact—if the matron does not object.

We may summarize the aims of a music program for a long-stay ward thus:

1. Encourage movement of the whole body by simple games and dances.

2. Encourage social interaction by talking about the music, why songs or records are chosen and what memories they bring back.

3. Encourage good breathing in singing to encourage lung ventilation and general physical and mental alertness.

4. Help patients to feel that their ideas are valuable, that they still have a status as individuals who matter in the world, even if physically they are unable to get around. There is a great deal of wisdom to be found in the thoughts and words of elderly patients, and we need not feel that we are being hypocritical in encouraging them to believe that their ideas are worth something.

Whether a music program will take place in ward or dayroom depends on circumstances—e.g. how ill the patients are and how much cooperation one can get from nursing staff to wheel invalid chairs or even beds around the hospital. The best situation is to have the music in a separate room, so that patients meet those from other rooms and wards and thus widen their social horizons. However, for the gravely ill, this may not be possible. In this case, a portable instrument must be used, with a brief session in each room. On no account should those in bed be ignored. They are all the more in need of stimulation, and should in some ways take priority over those who can walk.

REFERENCES

1. Exton-Smith, A. N. *Medical Annual of 1970;* Chapter on Geriatrics, John Wright, Bristol, 1970.
2. Newnham, W. H. 'Music therapy, tension and relaxation'; paper pub. by British Society for Music Therapy, 1964.
3. Boxberger, R. *et al.* 'The geriatric patient', in *Music in Therapy*, (ed.) Gaston, E., Macmillan, New York, 1968, p. 271.
4. Hirschberg, G., Lewis, L. and Thomas, D. *Rehabilitation*, Lippincott, Philadelphia, 1964, p. 360.
5. Blocker, W. P. and Gonzalez, F. R., 'Pulmonary exercises in obstructive pulmonary disease', *Journal of The American Geriatrics Society*, vol. XVIII, no. 8, 1970, pp. 615-622.
6. Critchley, McD. *The Parietal Lobes*, Arnold, London, 1963, p. 55.
7. Semmes, J. *et al.* 'Correlates of impaired orientation in personal and extrapersonal space', *Brain*, vol. 86, pt. 4, Dec. 1963, pp. 474-482.
8. Gerstmann, J. 'Some notes on Gerstmann's syndrome', *Neurology*, no. 7, Dec. 1957, pp. 866-9.
9. Critchley, McD. *op. cit.*, p. 203.
10. *Ibid.* p. 233.
11. Schreuder, J. Th. 'Hemiplaegia and its treatment', *Triangle 6*, Sandoz, 1964, p. 232.
12. Hirschberg, G., Lewis, L. and Thomas, D. *op. cit.*, p. 181.

13. *Equipment and staffing problems*

This section is mainly a summing up of suggestions and ideas already mentioned, together with a few possibilities which have not been described.

STAFF

In those parts of the world where music therapy is available as a professional career, it should be possible to employ a part or full-time therapist for a large geriatric unit who would lead all the activities, either in the planning or the actual work itself. However, for smaller units, such as nursing homes or smaller hospitals, or in the countries where there is no training in music therapy, some other course must be adopted.

1. There may be on the staff a musically minded occupational therapist or other staff member who would be interested and competent to direct a program of musical activity.

2. It may be possible to arrange for a local musician, either in an honorary or paid capacity, to undertake the work, with discussion among the medical and paramedical team as to what work should be undertaken.

3. A pianist could be employed purely as an accompanist, to provide music for exercises etc., the session being run by an occupational therapist, physiotherapist or social worker, depending on their individual interests and gifts.

4. A co-operative pianist could be asked to make tape recordings of suitable music for such exercises as are needed, and, when used in conjunction with 'sing-along' records (designed for people to join in and not merely listen to), this could be the basis of a reasonably satisfactory musical program. A tape recorder has several advantages over a 'live' musician. A taped accompaniment can be used for just a few moments, whereas one might hesitate to ask a pianist to play for such a short time. The volume of a taped accompaniment can be reduced very easily, thus allowing it to be placed very close to the patient, avoiding disturbance to

others. One could never do this with a piano. A compact tape recorder can also be taken where no piano could be fitted in.

EQUIPMENT

In a hospital which has good local support, it should be possible to obtain a piano, and if a good player-piano can be obtained, so much the better, since it will enable patients to make music for themselves. It has the added advantage of providing treadle-type exercise, which is beneficial for many patients whose leg musculature needs strengthening. Second-hand rolls of pianola music should be obtainable through an advertisement or a news paragraph in a district paper, and can also be bought in second-hand shops, at church fetes and so on. Modern rolls are still being cut, so that one is not restricted to old-fashioned music. (Even among the aged, there are some who like to hear the music of to-day, either because they feel it proves they are not as out-of-date as may be imagined, or because they genuinely like modern music, often after hearing it played by their grandchildren.)

For units where no piano can be obtained, the simple autoharp is a good substitute for social music activities, but less so for gymnastics, etc., because the tone is not as definite and firm as that of a piano. However, for some of the smooth-flowing work, such as head and neck movements, the softer tone would not matter. Different sized instruments are available, but all are of relatively modest cost.

A tape recorder is an essential for any serious program of music therapy. It should be one which has a good tape counter on it, so that small sections can be identified and selected without running through great lengths of tape. The recorder enables one to record band or orchestra work for criticism by the group, making it a more constructive activity than is otherwise possible. It can also be used in conjunction with a speech therapy program to enable patients to hear themselves singing and talking. In units where no accompanist is available, it can be used to prepare accompaniments for any session as required. There are many pianists in the community who could be persuaded to perform such a service for a hospital, because it could be done at leisure at a time which suited the pianist and not necessarily when the music would be in progress at the hospital—although ideally the pianist should observe one or two sessions in order to have an idea of what is required.

A portable instrument such as a guitar or piano accordion is most helpful in much hospital work. Because it is portable it can be taken from bed to bed in a ward; it can also be played directly in front of patients who are deaf, even right against the ear if necessary. Furthermore, it is played as one faces the patients and not, as with a piano, with one's back to them. By this, one attains a much better contact and sense of personal involvement.

In choosing band instruments, the therapeutic possibilities in aiding hand function should be remembered, but these are not the only considerations. Other factors to be remembered are the rhythmic use of the instruments, their use in aiding co-ordination, and also the aesthetic values. With suitable patients, it is possible to organise a combined occupational therapy program in which musical instruments are made for individuals or for the group. Books available for assistance in planning such an activity are the Penguin book, *Play with a Purpose for the Under 7s*, which has many ideas about improvising instruments, and two books published by Dryad Handicrafts, of Leicester, England. One of these is an inexpensive booklet about the making of recorders, and the other a bigger book called *Musical Instruments Made to be Played*. This has all the necessary details of materials, quantities, etc., with paper patterns of some instruments.

A possible collection of instruments would include: Cymbals of different sizes, down to those $1\frac{1}{2}$ inches in diameter, if possible; castanets on handles; castanets with elastic springs; bells on oval handles (usually called sleigh bells) to slip over knuckles; bells on stick handles; tambourines (small ones are suitable, and cheaper than those of large diameter); bongo drums; rhythm sticks, with painted bands of colour, for co-ordination work; xylophone or chime bars, for melodic work and for deaf patients; zither-type instrument, for melodic work and individual music-making.

The precise numbers needed of each instrument cannot be laid down; it can only be decided by the number of patients in a unit, what treatment they are having, how many patients will make up the music group and so on. The instruments listed above are all readily available, so it is not necessary to make a once-only decision as to what to buy. One can start with a small collection and add to it as necessary.

RECORD PLAYERS, PIPED MUSIC AND CHOICE OF RECORDS

A record player which is transportable from room to room has some advantages over the fixed type. Records can be played either as cheerful background music at meal times (when the concentration required for many disabled people to manage eating often precludes any conversation so that there is often a rather silent atmosphere) or specifically for listening. Any collection should be chosen with both purposes in mind. When facilities are available for piped music, cassettes will probably be used, but it is essential that there should be no monotony about the music played. So for piped music it is still more essential to have a generous supply of recordings available than is the case with ordinary records, in which it is easier to pick out a short excerpt from an LP.

The nucleus of a record collection might consist of: Background music such as the Melachrino Strings and Mantovani; Strauss waltzes; March tunes, old time dances (e.g. polkas, quadrilles) *played in strict tempo*; Sing-along (i.e. records for people to sing with, not to listen to); Popular classics; Christmas carols, preferably sung 'straight' so that patients may join in; Musical comedy numbers, such as 'White Horse Inn' and 'South Pacific'; Ballads, preferably with some Scottish songs, some Irish, and others depending on predominant nationality of patients in group; Sound-effects recordings, e.g. street noises, weather, children, etc. (Lists of such recordings will be found in any record catalogue); 'music for movement'.

If a system of sound reproduction is to be installed, the switching should be such as to allow flexibility so that it can be switched off in some rooms from the central switch, not an 'all on or all off' system. In addition, each room in which there is a speaker should have individual volume control, operated from the speaker, in case it is desired to have the sound louder in some rooms (e.g. where there is a number of profoundly deaf patients), and softer in others (where, perhaps, it is desired to have music as background only). It should also be planned so that a microphone can be used, for patients to present their own quasi-radio sessions, announcing the choices of different patients to give them a feeling of personal contact. Wisely used, a system of sound reproduction has almost infinite possibilities; used thoughtlessly, the boredom it can inflict—with consequent withdrawal—is endless.

In all planning of hospital music, one should never be afraid to be original and creative. We must improvise, invent, think ahead, but with humility enough to change our plans when the general good dictates this.

RECOMMENDED READING
Scott, M. M. *What Can I Play?* (3rd edn.), Benn, London, 1960.

Index